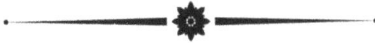

Living
BEYOND BURNOUT

Publisher

ENRICHED ENTERPRISES

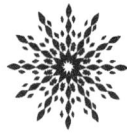

Living

BEYOND BURNOUT

❁

LISA MURRAY

First published in 2017 by Enriched Enterprises Pty Ltd
PO Box 2473, Noosa Heads, QLD, 4567, Australia
www.CreativeAlchemi.com
www.LivingBeyondBurnout.com
www.StopWaitingStartCreating.com
lisa@creativitylab.tv

National Library of Australia Cataloguing-In-Publication data:

Author:	Murray, Lisa
Title:	LIVING BEYOND BURNOUT
ISBN-13:	978-0-9942433-2-4
Subjects:	creativity, business, burnout, mindset, self-help, stress, fatigue, self-care, loving your work

Editor: Cassandra Russell
Internal Design: Anuradha Sen
Cover Design: Shayna Fernando
Front Cover Photography: Karen Cougan
Back Cover Photography: Pernilla Helmersson

BONUS RESOURCES:
www.CreativeAlchemi.com
www.LivingBeyondBurnout.com
www.LivingBeyondBurnout.com/inspire
www.LivingBeyondBurnout.com/Actions
www.LivingBeyondBurnout.com/Podcast
Www.LivingBeyondBurnout.com/quiz

DISCLAIMER:
This book is not intended to provide personalised health advice. Please ensure that you connect with appropriate healthcare practitioners for your situation. The authors and the publisher specifically disclaim any liability, loss or risk which is incurred as a consequence, directly or indirectly through the use and application of any contents of this work.

Any websites referenced in this book may change without notice.

DEDICATION

This book is dedicated to everyone who has ever had a breakdown, who ever felt like they were 'just holding it together', who has ever lost their mojo, or who has ever looked at their life and said 'there must be something better than this!'

Know that you are not alone, not the first and not the last to find the craziness of life on planet earth a little challenging. Most of all, know there is always something better if you are willing to embrace your brilliance… what other possibilities are you willing to choose?

ACKNOWLEDGMENTS

There are many people who deserve acknowledgment for the genesis of this book.

Firstly, my heartfelt thanks to Nicole Cody, life purpose intuitive and amazing inviter of possibilities. You were the first to show me the potency of me – you shone a spotlight on the entrance to a path I have had much joy in discovering!

Gary Douglas and Dr Dain Heer, co-creators of Access Consciousness®. Your tools were the catalyst that took me from burnout to owning way more of the potency of me and having the joy of generating multiple businesses without overwhelm. Thank you for allowing me to share just a little of the phenomenal magic that Access Consciousness offers.

The many business coaching clients I have worked with who, simply through being the amazing people they are, have shown me so much about what it means to be high achieving and aware and what phenomenal results are possible when these gifts are strategically applied. You know who you are. Every single one of you is phenomenal in your own special way! Thank you for inspiring this book and allowing your experiences to be shared with many others who will benefit.

My parents, for being there when I truly needed support. No words will ever be enough for the gratitude I have.

And lastly, the three furry friends who have kept me company during my intense bursts of writing this book. It has been nine years in the creating and there have been lots of cuddles, giggles and foot-warming moments along the way. Even though you are no longer with us, your magic is not forgotten.

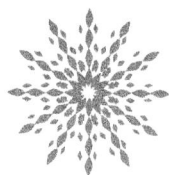

Contents

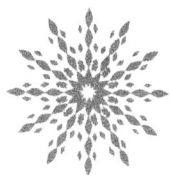

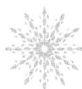

How to Read This Book
A Personal Hello!

Not a single person on this planet was born with burnout, yet there are hundreds of thousands of people trying to survive it every day. It's not natural. It's not normal. And it's time to change this situation.

When did we allow fatigue and exhaustion to become a normal part of working? When did we decide that everyone else's needs are more important than ours? When did we make the choice that over-delivering until we are so exhausted we can't move off the couch is still 'not enough'? The truth is, we've been sold a pack of lies about our true value in the world.

These are big questions that need to be asked at the very core of our society. As well as being a tool for preventing and transforming burnout, this book is your conversation starter for creating a kinder, more nurturing, more joy-filled future — in your work, your relationships and your life. Somewhere in the last couple of hundred years we collectively decided that work is more important than being healthy and energised. Over-working and over-giving don't work. Let's explore a range of different possibilities.

This is the book I tried not to write. For eight years. I didn't want to revisit the past. I am joyfully well. I am immersed in a collection of creative business projects and a marvellous new life. I get to play, and travel, and write and meet amazing kind, generous people. The B word was supposed to be a part of my past that stayed there, where it belonged. I discovered it is a stubborn little B. It wasn't happy with being swept under the carpet. It demanded I highlight it as a conversation the world must have. So here we are. Thank you for joining me. I'm sorry it is under these circumstances.

Let's be clear. I'm not sorry to be putting this conversation front and centre. No-one should have to live with burnout. It is totally preventable. And totally changeable. It doesn't have to evolve into chronic fatigue or fibromyalgia or depression. If you have burnout, you don't have to wrap yourself in cotton wool for the rest of your life. There is a way forward that is more energising and more fulfilling than the life you've known so far.

MY PERSONAL STORY

I had burnout three and a half times in 15 years. The first time I was 27, living in a big city that was uncompromisingly harsh on my highly sensitive nature, and working in a toxic environment. I didn't know it was burnout. I thought I couldn't cope and that I was a failure (because that's what I was told). So I ran away overseas for a couple of months, came back and continued my life as if nothing was wrong. I had no idea I'd already made a mess of my adrenals and that all of that stored trauma was sitting there waiting for Pandora's Box to open.

The next time I had burnout I was in my early thirties and working for a small business. The combination of unrelenting, unrealistic expectations and a nasty vindictive culture once again created immense exhaustion and a desperate need for change.

I left that job under less than happy circumstances, knowing within myself I'd delivered more than I'd promised, despite the unprofessional working conditions and the lack of gratitude for my contributions. By this time, I'd come to the conclusion that being tired was normal. That this was what my working life would be for the foreseeable future. I had completely forgotten how much I loved working in creative, playful ways. I'd completely forgotten my dreams of owning a business. I had no sense of how to enjoy my life if it didn't involve alcohol, hanging out with friends or playing with my dog. Moving jobs improved my day to day experience, but underneath it all, the unspoken, unacknowledged B word silently lurked, stealthily plotting another turn in the spotlight.

During the next years, I chose to have a series of what I call 'holiday jobs', where I shut down my brilliance and did jobs that were easy, so that I could find a different way forward. That worked wonderfully well until I couldn't keep my capabilities a secret any longer. I was offered jobs with more responsibility and in so many ways I loved them. I was creating on a much bigger scale and leading change in meaningful ways. There was a blissful interlude where I had a boss who was presence, peace and calm in action. He was brilliant, capable and he didn't do hustle. I thought I'd found nirvana. We were a great team and I was hugely disappointed when I had to give that job back to its owner after a couple of years.

Having regained my confidence, I took on a huge job in the same organisation. It was horrendous. We were hugely under-staffed and under-resourced and there was an enormous amount of infighting and undermining between the different silos that were supposed to be changing the world together. Every day brought a new set of issues which seemed to have little resolution as people doggedly held onto their turf wars. This was eye-opening for me. I was interested in creating a greater future for the world, not fighting for budgets and territories. Yes, you can call me naive. At the same time, I had an uncanny knack for naming the elephant in the room, much to the discomfort of many around me. It wasn't a comfortable time for anyone.

To escape the incessant insanity and bring the energy of creativity into my life, I started an MBA and began overseeing a house renovation. Within 18 months I was so far into burnout territory that this time I knew I had to discover its name. Strike three, I was out! This recurrent pattern had to stop. I inelegantly fell to pieces as the B word launched a full-scale attack on my body. I cried in my office. Sometimes I napped just to get through the day. Even after a month off work, I couldn't stay out of bed for more than a few hours, or verbalise a coherent sentence. The enormous and unrelenting stress had fried a whole lot of circuits in my body and brain. I quit my job, a shell of my true self. And I wondered how I would get better. It was the worst of times and one of the greatest gifts of my life.

At that time, I didn't know what self-care was. I didn't know I'd snuffed out the flame of my brilliance by believing the non-stop judgement. I had forgotten what my creative flow felt like. And I was insane enough to imagine that having a few months off would fix everything. That was not exactly how it panned out.

The story of my recovery is contained within this book. As I was writing, a burnout prevention model evolved. This model is the base for a simple system for prevention and recovery. I didn't live it in a linear way, however it is written so that you have the choice to discover the elements that will create the most change for you. This system is a more useful way forward for you than the boring nitty gritty of my 'day in - day out' story. My recovery time would have been substantially shorter than the two years it took, had anyone been talking about burnout in these ways at the time. The years of trial and error, experiments and adventures are now my gift to you.

Oh yes... the half. When I recovered from the severe burnout, I had the bright idea of starting a relationship. It didn't go well. He is a narcissist. I am an empath. There's never a happy ending in that situation. When I left him, I was exhausted and on the edge of collapse from the daily abuse that was projected at me. Fortunately, by this time, I'd discovered some great tools for changing my physical, mental and emotional states. I recovered faster than ever before and did the inner work around my not-so-cool habit of attracting abusive people into my life. That could be the subject of another book. For now I'll just say that toxic people won't mess with you when you own your power and potency, and when you show up as the brilliance you truly are.

Fast forward to now and I have a beautiful, imperfect, ever-changing life. One that nurtures and nourishes me, one that allows me to be that inspired, creative change-leader I was so desperately seeking to be back in 2009. Yes, there have been many ups and downs along the way, and I wouldn't change where I am now for any amount of financial 'security' and overwork.

Thank you for reading my story. Please know that your story may be different and your experience of it is what it is. This book is an invitation to discover a new way forward. You don't have to read it from start to finish. Take what talks to you in your current situation and leave the rest until it calls you. Your recovery is like a treasure map rather than a superhighway. Enjoy this journey, it will nourish and inspire you long after the burnout is gone.

HOW TO READ THIS BOOK

Most books don't need to explain themselves. This one wants to. Mostly because if you read it when you are deep in burnout, you may find it to be more than you need in any single specific moment. When you have burnout, the most ease-filled way forward is one choice at a time. Right now, you may only need to read a page or two at a time. You don't need the masterplan all at once, (unless you love a helicopter view) and I wanted to ensure it is all here for you for when you are ready.

If there is a chapter that sounds like a foreign language, just know that it is not for you right now. I've shared eight years of dynamic change with you in less than 210 pages. You will grow, evolve and discover in the timing and ways that are natural to your life. Don't try to force yourself to have it all now. Allow the changes to unfold as they can. This is a book you'll be able to read again ten years from now and still discover something new!

The Burnout Breakthrough Model includes 4 elements: change and choice; nurture and nourishment; creative energy and brilliance. If one of these topics talks to you, start with those chapters. Or you can just ask your body a question 'what do you know about what we need right now?', and then open the book up randomly. You'll find your own way forward.

Burnout Breakthrough Actions offer simple ways for getting started by doing something different. There are one or two in each chapter and they are highlighted in their own box.

Pause. Breathe. Pages are a resting space. An invitation to stop, smell the roses and be kind to you. When you come to one, don't rush past it, give yourself a few minutes to indulge in the space of there being nothing you need to do.

Inspiration and Insights Pages are a space for noting your aha moments, for writing sweet notes to yourself, for highlighting what you are going to do different.

The *Fearless First Aid* chapter is a great place to start if you are desperately seeking symptomatic relief.

The change you are seeking doesn't have a recipe. It's an adventure in (re)discovering the magic of your life. As you read this book, be kind to you. Don't force it. Allow yourself to be present with the new ways of living it offers. If what you have been doing would fix your situation, we wouldn't be sharing this conversation. Every tiny choice is a valuable choice. Whether it makes a difference instantly or not. The effects of the choices offered in these pages are cumulative.

What kind of life do you truly desire to live? Your body has shown you it is time to make new choices. Gather up your courage, allow your energy to build, and enjoy the journey.

WHO IS THIS BOOK FOR?

This book is especially for the amazing over-committed, over-achievers (ahem, workaholics!) who may also be empathic or highly sensitive. These people are highly susceptible to exhaustion, burnout and hiding their true brilliance. Empaths and highly sensitive people over-give; workaholics and over-achievers over-work (surprise!) and over-deliver to prove their value.

These personality traits are more susceptible to burnout because they include gifts that are easily crushed or disregarded in the density and heaviness of how it 'should be' in this reality. What if we know of different and greater possibilities? Is it time to acknowledge that there is more than one way to create - that it's not all about the hustle or being insanely productive?

This book is also designed for coaches, therapists, mentors, managers and leaders... It's the book I would have loved to have when I started coaching. It's also the book I wish my managers had read before they tried to squash me into a box that I just didn't fit into, no matter how much I contorted myself to fit their expectations.

If you are a leader, I ask you to consider if it is time for a new way of leading sensitive people. Those who are sensitive have (often unconsciously) put up such huge protective barriers and behaviours to manage their sensitivity in harsh environments, that others perceive them as insensitive. These highly sensitive people are some of your most brilliant team members. Do you truly desire to lose their gifts and contributions? Or does it make more sense to find ways for your workplace to work with those capacities in different ways? What would be possible if we could all look beyond the conclusions and assumptions that are commonly made?

This book shares with you the journey I took, and the practical, life-changing tools I have discovered and explored with many of my inspirational business coaching clients — each of them wonderful, over-achieving, acutely aware, amazing beings in their own individual ways!

PAUSE. BREATHE.

BE.

A GIFT FOR YOU

In closing my personal message to you, I offer you this love note…

Dear YOU,

The B word can be one of the greatest gifts of your life if you will allow it to show you a new way forward. The old ways are no longer viable. Together we are creating a new world. A world where kindness to self and others prevails. A world where money is enjoyed, but it is not the driving force. A world where you can be you and enjoy this magical thing we call living.

Thank you for finding your way to this book. Thank you for reading it with an open, curious mind and a heart full of vulnerability. Thank you for showing your body that you adore it, and that your relationship with it is going to change.

Know this:

> Burnout rarely visits the weak and easily lead.
>
> You are much more magnificent than you imagine.

Be daring. Be kind. Be present.

These are the magic wands you are seeking.

You have everything you need.

Lisa Murray

P.S. You may be resisting the idea that you have burnout... I get it! I did too. Don't let that stop you from using these ideas and strategies to have more energy and more joy than you've ever had before... Over to you!

FOUR ELEMENTS FOR
LIVING BEYOND BURNOUT

During the creation of this book many people asked me for a list of symptoms that would allow them to avoid burnout. It is clear to me that once you've started being aware of the symptoms, it's mostly too late to stop burnout from starting. Your body is already giving you the signals loud and clear. That list will come later, right now I'd rather give you this. A simple recipe for preventing burnout by making choices that bring you alive.

There are four essential elements that will allow you to avoid burnout and live magnificently. These same four elements will transform your burnout into a breakthrough. They are the basis of this book so we'll be talking about them in much more detail in future chapters.

1. A willingness to change.

2. A deeply nurturing, nourishing life.

3. Exploration and expression of your creative energies.

4. The liberation of your brilliance.

As you use each of these elements to bring yourself alive, you will amplify your energy in your life and the world.

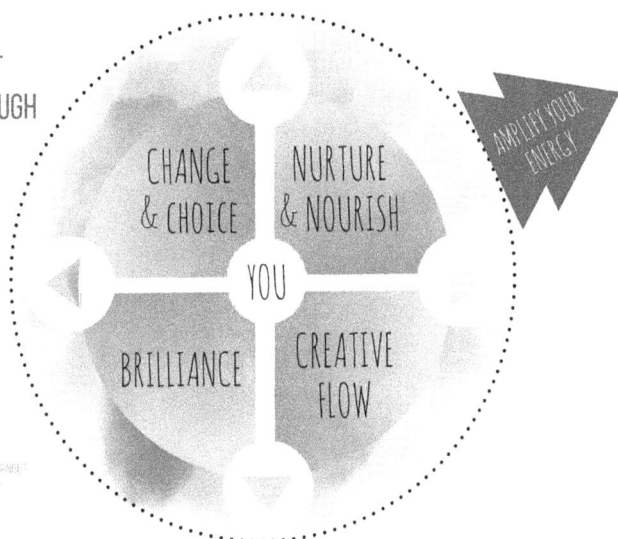

BURNOUT
BREAKTHROUGH
MODEL

CHANGE & CHOICE

NURTURE & NOURISH

YOU

BRILLIANCE

CREATIVE FLOW

AMPLIFY YOUR ENERGY

These elements can also be explored as questions. If you do nothing but ask these four questions and respond to the awareness you receive, your exhaustion will begin to change.

Even now, whenever I sense even a twinge of tiredness, these are my go to questions:

1. Is this the change I have been asking for, showing up in unexpected ways?

2. What is the nurture and nourishment that will make the greatest difference to me right now?

3. Is there a more creative possibility available?

4. Is my brilliance stifled or depressed in some way?

Logic cannot answer these questions accurately. Your willingness to be present and allow new insights to come will offer different choices for your future. Are you open to living a greater life?

If you'd like to know which of these elements is most relevant for you right now, take the *Amplify Your Energy Quiz at www.LivingBeyondBurnout.com/quiz* It will show you which of the 4 elements from the Burnout Breakthrough Model will make the greatest difference to you immediately. Ultimately you'll benefit from playing with all four elements, and it's great to have a place to start. You can retake the quiz as your life changes and it will lead you through each of the elements in the ideal sequence for you.

BURNOUT
BREAKTHROUGH ACTION

Throughout this book, I'll offer simple ways to start unravelling the junk-fuelled choices that are feeding your burnout like sugar on steroids. If you play with them, you'll uncover what started your burnout and what can change it.

Burnout seems to appear out of nowhere. And yet its roots start growing months and years in advance of the symptoms bursting onto the scene. Burnout starts with our over-thinking mind, and that never-ending demand of ourselves to *do* more — for ourselves and others. It starts with every thought that says "I should…", "I must…", "I have to…".

ACTION

For the next 24 hours, write down every thought you have that starts with "I should…", "I must…", "I have to…". Tick off the ones that you act on.

Are your action items a great match to what you truly desire? Or are you deep in perfection or people-pleasing territory?

Within this list are the seeds of your burnout, stealthily growing stronger and more dominant with every tiny action that isn't resonant with the true you.

INSPIRATION
& INSIGHTS

SECTION
I

BURNOUT?
How Did I Get Here?

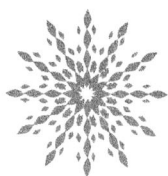

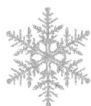

Are You Living With Burnout?

DOES BURNOUT HAVE YOU IN ITS NEEDY CLUTCHES?

"How do I know if I have burnout?" is one of the most common questions I hear. The answer depends on who you listen to. In the *Amplify Your Energy Lounge* I talk to a wide range of people who treat burnout in different ways, and who work with different physical, emotional and psychological signals for identifying burnout. Confusion is common as many of these symptoms may also be indicative of other diagnoses as well. If it was easy to define, I wouldn't have had to write this book!

The first two times I had burnout, I was not treated for burnout, simply because I didn't know that's what was going on. Back then, there was little awareness of burnout and people presenting with those symptoms were treated for depression or as if they were having a breakdown. Neither of which are entirely accurate.

The early signals of burnout are that subtle phase where you brush everything off as 'I'm just tired' or 'I'm going through a busy patch' or 'When X changes, I'll be happier and less stressed'. Here's the thing, if you aren't full of joy, energy and a desire to live full out in every area of your life, you may be sitting on the edge of a mild case of burnout. If everything is an effort and you're constantly exhausted or you're having mini (or maxi) meltdowns, you've moved a little beyond the mild case into more full-blown symptoms.

What are the symptoms of burnout? You have no 'get up and go'. Your body will not move, even when you will it to. You fixate on emergencies, resentments, problems, catastrophising and your doctor may have decided you are depressed, but you know the anti-depressants aren't changing anything, they're just masking your symptoms.

Maybe you feel unsupported, unrewarded, unacknowledged and overworked. Your joy got sucked down the toilet months ago. You're cynical, defensive and emotionally drained. You can't sleep and it's not because you're way too excited about living!

Physically you may be experiencing adrenal fatigue, weight changes, digestive issues and intense aches and pains - or in more extreme cases be diagnosed with stress-related illnesses such as chronic fatigue syndrome, heart disease or fibromyalgia. If you're relying on stimulants, they no longer give you the energy you're seeking.

Mentally you may have memory loss, incoherence, and your mind... Just. Won't. STOP! All you ever talk about is what's wrong. You're marginally functional and mostly at the effect of uncontrollable emotional intensity, which may show up as crying every time you turn around or losing your shit over what would normally be mildly annoying inconveniences. If you're an introvert, it's likely you are completely removing yourself from any kind of non-essential contact with people.

All of these choices are signals that your systems are overloaded and your normal coping mechanisms have shut down. You're in a rut if these are fairly new symptoms; you have burnout if you've been experiencing them for months or years or you've blown a few circuits that you can't get working again.

If any of these symptoms sound even slightly familiar, it's time to make different choices, even if you haven't got enough energy to raise your middle finger right now. How messy do you have to get before you change your reality? You can listen to the whispers, or you can wait for the sledgehammer of exhaustion to fell you in a king-hit that lands you in a deep, dark crevice, where the only way left is up.

THE 12 STAGES OF BURNOUT :: SYMPTOMS

Psychologists Herbert Freudenbürger and Gail North created a twelve stage model that identifies a wide variety of symptoms, which may exist simultaneously and/or in a different order to what is presented here. Treatment may begin at any of these stages and is commonly based on symptomatic relief. Without addressing the self-worth points of view which underly the need to prove yourself, progress can be slower and smaller than you desire.

THE FREUDENBÜRGER AND NORTH MODEL:

1. A compulsion to prove yourself.
2. Working harder without switching off.
3. Neglecting your needs.
4. Displacing conflicts and dismissing problems.
5. Revising values and favouring work over everything.
6. Denying emerging problems and being intolerant.
7. Withdrawing from life.
8. Odd behavioural changes.
9. Depersonalising and devaluing self and other people.
10. Inner emptiness filled by addictions.
11. Depression.
12. Total mental and physical collapse.

Even in environments with extreme demands, burnout begins with a need to prove your worth, which leads to working harder, which leads to neglecting your needs for wellbeing. This is the start of the slippery slope. Conflicts and problems are ignored and anxiety and panic can set in. These symptoms can be present whether your burnout is caused by a personal or professional situation. Abusive relationships are triggered by the same self-worth issues, with the added burden of living in an unsafe home environment.

Work (or the relationship) becomes the only focus as you try to deliver to impossible (often self-imposed) standards. In some workplaces this is caused by unrealistic expectations. In an abusive relationship, it can be caused by consistent gas-lighting by your narcissistic boss, partner or friend. People with healthy boundaries and a clear sense of self will find a different way forward. For those who love to meet expectations, those boundaries disappear with alarming ease.

As you work harder, you deny emerging problems and become increasingly intolerant of colleagues, family and friends. These interpersonal conflicts often lead to social withdrawal and an increasing dependence on drugs and alcohol. At this point, friends and family may be concerned about the behaviour changes, but the person exhibiting them does not see a problem. This is where the issue has become depersonalised - no-one, including the person with the symptoms, is seen as valuable, and the needs for thrival are not met.

As the burnout sufferer's wellbeing takes a nose-dive, an inner emptiness emerges that is band-aided with addictions — to food, sex, alcohol, exercise or living online. These habits ensure that the future looks bleak and dark and the addictions feed the feelings of exhaustion, leading to a sense of depression. At this point the person is not functioning in their brilliance and is most likely not performing well at work.

As the pressure mounts, it leads to full burnout — a total mental and physical collapse that requires an intervention. The burnout breakthrough model we will be exploring in this book includes lifestyle changes, the choice to nurture and nourish the body in new ways, an immersion in creative energies to refresh the spirit, and the willingness to work only in your zone of brilliance.

PAUSE. BREATHE.

RELAX.

ALTERNATIVE BURNOUT MODEL :: CATALYSTS & CAUSES

Personal experience and my work with people who have burnout has uncovered another way burnout is triggered. If you've experienced a big change or choice that on the surface looks wonderful, but doesn't match where you truly need to be in life, your spirit lets you know by sending you the gift of physical burnout, so that you cannot pursue that which is not a great fit for you. This kind of burnout occurs because your life force is being suffocated by choices that don't resonate with who you truly are. It's the absence of being you.

My Burnout Catalyst Model:

1. Catalyst = a new 'good' choice that isn't working for you.

2. Subtle physical and emotional hints go unnoticed or are ignored.

3. Symptoms intensify and surface level treatments are applied.

4. Symptoms re-occur once surface level treatments stop.

5. Catalyst is identified / burnout is acknowledged.

6. Resistance to change emerges (fear, shame, survival issues).

7. Major health crisis / inability to continue on current path.

8. Change is identified and chosen. Your transformation begins.

9. Intensive nurture and nourishment of ALL of you.

10. Creative energies are liberated. Brilliance is expressed. Burnout disappears.

Steps 3 and 4 can be avoided if you listen to the subtle changes in Step 2.

Step 6 and 7 can be prevented if you are willing to embrace the change your spirit is demanding immediately, rather than resisting.

Are you wondering if this is you? This is how it looks when you're living it:

You make an exciting new choice. As the gloss of your new adventure wears off and what was fun turns into obligation, your body starts to offer subtle hints that this isn't going well. You brush them off as low-grade tiredness or misery that will pass any day now. Except that if nothing changes, those symptoms move into a slow, steady decline. These symptoms are often managed via surface level 'self-care' fixes for the body that don't change the underlying situation. For example, getting a massage or taking vitamins.

These mini-fixes and temporary solutions make little long-term difference and at some point, the person finds their symptoms have intensified to such a degree that they cannot be ignored. At this point, you may go on stress leave or have recurrent physical symptoms that leave you more and more exhausted. Chronic health conditions can set in.

Acknowledging that you have burnout can be a major turning point, or a major source of resistance. If it is a turning point, you'll seek both treatment and transformation and your life will become much more enjoyable sooner!

If you resist the diagnosis, you'll prolong the suffering until it almost kills you. (Please don't feel bad if this is where you are right now, I've been there and you can live a wonderful life beyond burnout… keep reading!!)

The refusal to change often shows up as trying harder and working more, as if you are not doing enough already. Underneath is a sense of shame and embarrassment because of the failure of having to admit you are not coping. This can also trigger fear and survival issues, with 'but....' featuring often in your conversations. I remember saying to my acupuncturist 'but why can't I work from bed?' I loved my work a lot more than my body, which was a true unkindness!

If you hold firm to your resistance an unambiguous trigger point will arrive in the form of major health issues or the inability to perform your work. It will feel like you have no choice. In reality, you have ignored the thousands of choice points that have been tugging at you for months or years. You don't have to wait for a tipping point to make the change that your life and body are asking of you!

As soon as you become willing to choose again, your transformation can begin. Your breakthrough is realised through the four elements we discussed at the start of the book. We will delve deeper into each one as this book progresses. Remember, you don't have to read this book linearly. If one of these topics is talking to you right now, go there!

1. Embracing change and inviting new choices.

2. Nurturing and nourishing the real you.

3. Liberating your creative energies.

4. Unleashing your brilliance and loving your work.

As you move through each of these stages, you become unstoppable. Instead of being irresistible to burnout, you repulse it, simply by being you. You are able to live a vibrant, fulfilling life, without constantly worrying about your energy levels. You'll have energy for more projects than you imagine possible. I know it sounds wildly improbably right now. I remember wondering if I was ever going to be able to work again. There is light at the end of this tunnel... and it is powered by your willingness to do something different!

PAUSE. BREATHE.

ALLOW.

PREVENTING BURNOUT

In hindsight, I'm aware I was living both models concurrently. The lethal combination of low self-worth (hello Little Ms Oversensitive), and making choices which I quietly and secretly sensed were not working for me, created a furnace with a huge supply of fuel for fanning the burnout flames. Leaving that fire unattended did more than singe my self-confidence. It almost burnt me to death.

If you'd like to prevent burnout (or stop it from reappearing), begin by questioning and identifying where you may currently be at risk. Is there anything in either of these models that are ringing fire alarms? Are there any smoke signals that you're ignoring because you have decided it's going to rain any moment and the risk of an out-of-control bushfire will be magically averted?

Do a little stocktake of your current situation. What needs to change? There's no shame in changing everything if it's going to create a life far greater than the one you have now. Even if your choices look totally crazy on the surface. You know. Trust yourself.

This is a time to be kinder to you than you've ever been.

A time to receive all the support people are offering you. A time to ask for what you need as you move towards living well and living vibrantly as the real you. Burnout burns all pretence away. Don't let it get that far. Drop everything that is not truly you and begin embracing the essence of your true brilliance and creative energies. From this space, everything becomes possible! I promise you won't regret the choice to put you first.

If you are a leader and you'd like to prevent burnout with your team, start by having open discussions about what burnout is and what the symptoms are. Identify 'at risk' team-members and work collaboratively with them to create the change that is required.

Most of all, put people first. Be like USA based CEO, Ben Congleton, who responded to his team-member's email about taking a mental health day off with this:

"I use (your email) as a reminder of the importance of using sick days for mental health – I can't believe this is not standard practice at all organisations. You are an example to us all, and help cut through the stigma so we can all bring our whole selves to work."

Her screen-shot of his response went viral on Twitter (over 16 000 shares and 45000 likes at the time of writing). This is a sad indicator of how rarely organisations support the people who support them. Imagine if this could be a 'normal' response in the majority of workplaces. How different would our world be?

Burnout is a wake-up call for the corporate world, for healthcare organisations and for entrepreneurs obsessed with hustle. It's a catalyst for organisations to begin to treat their people differently. It's an invitation for leaders to be an example of living and working in their creative brilliance, rather than forcing outcomes at any cost. This is not an individual problem. It is a collective and systematic societal issue that can be changed by being present with each other as people first. Living is a precious gift. No amount of money compensates for the death of your spirit.

One more thing. People will not even look at whether they have burnout if your organisation penalises them for this kind of illness by attacking their performance. If a staff member has a performance issue, consider whether burnout is partially or fully causing it. Not only did my boss save up all my work for when I got back from my month of stress leave; he also insisted on me having a 360-degree performance review at the height of my burnout. Those choices were unkind, unproductive and lead to intensified health issues, rather than resolving the underlying workload issues.

Your job as a leader is to inspire the best from your people, not to make them wrong. Being aware of the different choices available for creating new paths forward is the sign of a true leader. What questions can you ask that will lead to greater possibilities for everyone? What changes can you make that will allow your team to be in the right jobs, nurtured, nourished, creatively contributing and expressing their full brilliance?

If you are a leader on the edge of burnout, look at where you are over-giving or over-protective, or doing work that isn't yours to do. The change starts with you. If you don't know what to change, please get a coach who understands both burnout and how organisations work. It will be worth so much more than you pay!

Your health is priceless. The health of your organisation is priceless. Treat them that way.

BURNOUT
BREAKTHROUGH ACTION

As you read through this chapter, did you find yourself nodding your head in recognition? Or maybe squirming uncomfortably with the realisation that you aren't functioning at your best?

> Which stage/s of the Freudenbürger and North model are most true for you right now?

> Where are you living on the Burnout Catalyst model?

Your burnout can be a springboard into being everything you are, or a straitjacket that limits your choices for the rest of your life. That choice rests with you.

> What choice can you make that can bring wellness fully into your world?

> What is your next step?

> Physical first aid?

> Or liberating the real you?

If you are a leader, did any of this give you an aha that can open more authentic conversations with your team around this topic? Where will you start?

P.S. If you are seeking support with this process, there is a range of resources, services and programs available for individuals and organisations at www.LivingBeyondBurnout.com

INSPIRATION
& INSIGHTS

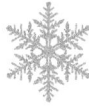

FEARLESS FIRST AID

You're exhausted. You know you need fast and
fearless first aid. Where do you start?

We all love instant relief, but treating your symptoms doesn't
stop the need to make bigger changes. Symptomatic relief gives
you the energy and enthusiasm to move towards sustainable
changes more easily. Please use these ideas to feel better; don't
neglect the trigger points that are showing you a more resonant
way forward. If you do, you'll negate the gift of burnout and it
will become the gift that keeps on giving you curry!

Please know that you are totally responsible for the choices
you make. These are suggestions that have worked for me at different times. They may or may not work in the same way for you.
Do your research. Ask questions. Listen to your body. You will
notice that I have not included standard medical treatments here.
I do not personally support the common approach to treat symptoms with drugs for depression due to the many side-effects and
addiction risks. Of course, you are free to, and should, make your
own choices.

SUPER STRATEGIES

These strategies can change multiple symptoms at once. Ask
your body what it is most drawn to and start there! They are not
'one-off' solutions and in most cases you will need to choose a
program of treatment.

1. Access Bars® — this was the work that made a huge difference
   to me physically, after a year of trying many different

modalities and therapists. Bars® is an energetic tool used for releasing trauma, exhaustion, overwhelm and much more. Based on the idea that your point of view creates your reality, it is a gentle, nurturing, hands-on-head energy process that dissipates the thoughts, feelings and emotions that keep your symptoms in place and stop you from making new choices. I had my Bars® run every week for a year and within the first three months, most of the physical symptoms permanently disappeared. There are thousands of practitioners world-wide. Find out more at www.AccessConsciousness.com/Bars.

2. Adrenal Fatigue and Nervous System Regulation — many people with burnout have a disregulated nervous system as a result of constant and prolonged stress. Your adrenals give you energy for living. When you are living in ways that don't support your aliveness, your adrenals know it. They are kind enough to say 'no, there's no energy for that!' as a way of giving you awareness that you have different ways forward. When you start trusting your body's awareness rather than berating it for not keeping up, you rediscover what living truly is for you.

Healing modalities that can assist with adrenal fatigue and nervous system issues include somatic psychotherapy, Chinese medicine, Ayurvedic treatments, acupuncture, flower essences, homeopathy, some forms of chiropractic, nutrition and diet, as well as physical exercise.

SPECIFIC SUPPORT STRATEGIES

TOOLS FOR EMOTIONAL SUPPORT

ANXIETY AND OVERWHELM:: A little high quality salt (e.g. Himalayan salt) under the tongue is great for anxiety and feeling scattered and unable to focus.

STRESS OR ANXIETY:: Bring your tongue down to rest at the bottom of your mouth to balance your autonomic nervous system. Breathe in and count to 6 and breathe out and count to 6 without any pauses in between the breaths. Breathe like this until you are calmer.

FOREST BATHING :: Spend a full day in a forest. Allow yourself to receive the healing that the trees offer. The Japanese call it shinrin-yoku and research has proven a wide variety of benefits.

TOOLS FOR PHYSICAL SUPPORT ::

SENSORY ENERGY BOOSTERS

SMELL:: A couple of drops of peppermint oil on the floor of a warm shower in the mornings will give you a delicious and energising aromatherapy wakeup. Finish off with a burst of cold water to get your cells singing, if you can brave it!

TASTE:: Nuts are a great energiser when you haven't got time to eat well. Low GI and full of goodness… get yourself a delicious nut mix and have a small handful whenever you feel your energy flagging. Cashews are a great anti-depressant and almonds are great for lowering blood pressure. Adding slivers of raw organic dark chocolate will make your nuts feel like a really blissful treat! Or you can eat nut butter with banana and strawberries for a decadent healthy snack. Too easy!

TOUCH:: Salt water is a very simple way to clear off lots of old energy and feel fresh and new again! An early morning trip to the beach or a good soak in an epsom salt bath or rubbing transdermal magnesium on your joints will see your energy rise and offer ease for your achy body.

SOUND:: Meditative music or visualisations are great for refreshing the spirit, as is a little Mozart. Sit yourself in a quiet dark room for 30 minutes with some soothing listening and you'll find yourself ready for the next round of celebratory cheer!

SIGHT:: Each of us has something that is mesmerising to our eyes... for me it is watching the ocean roll in, wave after wave. For others it is the flickering flame of a fire or candle. Whatever your version of mesmerising bliss is, give yourself at least 30 minutes to enjoy it and forget about everything else. Your sanity will soon return!!

TOOLS FOR MENTAL SUPPORT

STOP BEING OVER-STIMULATED:: A simple way to do this is to sit or lie in a dark room with no stimulation for at least 20 minutes. No music, no books, no podcasts, no lights. Just you and the room. Peace. Silence. Bliss. (And maybe it will be uncomfortable at first... after a while you'll love it!)

STOP OVER-THINKING:: Speed-write by dumping all your thoughts into a notebook is great (write by hand, not computer). As you write each thought, tell it that it is safe there and it doesn't need to come back into your head again. (And you don't need to re-read all that stuff again either!)

TOOLS FOR ENLIVENING YOUR SPIRIT

GIFT YOURSELF AN ELECTRONICS SABBATICAL:: When was the last time you disconnected from the world? Give yourself an hour or a day without electronics. Minimise the over-stimulation and allow yourself space to be present with people instead of keypads.

BE CREATIVE:: Exhaustion can be diminished by being creative in ways that allow your brain to have a holiday... Design your play for the energy level you have e.g. colouring in, finger-painting, play-doh... it's about losing yourself in the moment, not the results.

BAREFOOT BLISS:: Place your bare feet or entire body on the earth (even if it's cold!) for at least 10 - 15 minutes. This allows your body to connect with the planet, rather than running everything through your head. Mix it up while you're playing. Watch a sunrise or sunset. Pat a dog. Admire some flowers. Put your feet in the ocean, on some lovely smooth rocks or in the midst of an herb garden.

Tools for Changing Your Environment

Change up your workspace:: Where do you most love working? With a view or in a quiet space with no interruptions? What if it could be different everyday? What would nurture your body today?

I always ask my body where it would like to create today. Adding diversity to your work spaces allows the inspiration to flow continually. Sit next to different people. Work in the lunchroom or a different office. Take your work to a coffee shop or a co-working space. I like to write overlooking the beach.

Hold walking meetings:: Sitting still increases depression. When you walk and talk, however slowly you might move, your body gets to rearrange and dissipate stuck energy. If possible hold your meetings outside. Fresh air has magic in it!

Tools for Changing Your Priorities

Ditch your 'to-do' list:: If I'm following a to-do list, that is the space of least inspiration. When I follow my awareness of what is required to move forward with ease, inspiration comes with ease. What would work even better for you than a to-do list? I have a 'to-create' list that is a fall-back if I just can't come up with something that is fun for me to create. It doesn't have deadlines. It offers a creative mix of possibilities and adventures that have broad blisslines to keep me moving forward.

Pause. Breathe.

BE CURIOUS.

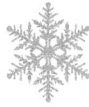

LIBERATING THE REAL YOU

Burnout is an invitation to liberate who you truly are.

You're not just a mother, a leader, a worker, a healer, a partner... you are a being with infinite possibilities that you haven't yet chosen. Exhaustion, stress and burnout are your wake-up calls. Are you going to choose a different future? Or will you insist on trying to create the same life you've been leading, sticky-taping over your symptoms and allowing your spirit to quietly die on the inside?

Do you remember baby pictures of you? Were you the cutest thing you've ever seen? Were you happy? Cuddly? Playful? That you was closer to the real you than you've been in a long time. We're not taking you back to baby land, but we are going to create a space where you can be even more happy, cuddly and playful than you remember!

Your breakthrough starts with embracing the void. It expands when you find your mojo. It stays when you make the changes your life is asking of you. Receive the nurturing your body desires. Immerse yourself in your creative energies. Allow your brilliance to dazzle the world.

THE VOID

Before the breakthrough comes the void. The void is the space of stillness and silence that you have been resisting as if your life depends on it.

You are juggling thousands of worries... thousands of things you are caring for... thousands of priorities... and none of them include you. All those worries, priorities and responsibilities need someone to love them. You feel like the entire world will fall apart if it isn't you. The bad news is, you are replaceable. The good news is, you are replaceable.

When I embraced the void, everything I imagined would fall apart without me began to come together in greater ways. People stepped up. Priorities were rearranged or discarded. New ways forward were forged. And I did not have to be the central pivot point of control anymore... which left a void. The void. The void I'd been avoiding as if I would die of it. The void that removes the residues of overwhelm and over-stimulation as a wave clears footsteps from the shore.

In truth, having an energised, nurturing life depends on embracing the void instead of the overwhelm. The void is a space where you get to let down your guard and allow yourself to be. In the beginning, it can be intensely uncomfortable as all of that external stimulation takes a back seat.

The ocean shows us the beauty of the void. It rolls to its own rhythms, never doubting its next wave. Never seeking a wave from a different shore. The ocean knows its bliss. When you watch the ocean rolling, hear the waves crashing in perfect timing, you sense the potent magic within these rhythms.

All your trying, all your striving, all your wishing, all your neediness shrinks from your mind and floats out to sea... leaving in its wake the essence of what you are here for. The liberation of the treasure of you. The bliss of being truly, deeply, wildly alive. It starts with the void.

Everything else is random debris. Entertaining for a moment. Important only because you've made it so. Relevant by your submission to a world that values doing over being. Made into mountains that must be climbed by your choice.

Being present with the void starts the process of unwinding the over-stimulation that keeps burnout alive. You suffocate the flame by removing the one thread that feeds the fire. The thread that will allow the intensity to unravel. It starts with doing less, not more. And in case you are having a mild panic right now, know this: the space you are entering isn't a dull void; it's a generative, creative, nurturing space that is waiting to invite you to new possibilities.

What is that one thread? For me it can be a few hours at the beach by myself, lying on the earth, listening to the waves and the birds. Not doing anything. Or it can be found in the magic of being with horses. Allowing them to contribute their energy in peaceful, gentle ways. It can also be found in making art for the pleasure of it, without any target in mind, without any judgement of the results. It can also be found in releasing the fascia in the body. Fascia is a network of connective tissue just beneath the skin that holds our body together in magical ways. Releasing it brings a sense of euphoria and space. Yin Yoga and Bowen Therapy are simple ways to start releasing your fascia.

You'll find your own ways of pulling the thread. Don't overthink it. Your body knows. Allow it to lead the way. When you pull the thread, your sensory awareness expands and you have the pleasure of losing your mind and embodying ALL that you are. In that space of being is the beginning of bliss.

At first the void seems extremely uncomfortable. There's just you… and You… and YOU. No distractions, no stimulation, no doing because you should, no answering to anyone else, no electronics. That raw blank canvas can be intimidating. It's tempting to fill it with busyness — anything to stop the silence that makes it obvious that you don't know or like you nearly as much as you could.

On the other side of the void is the breakthrough you are seeking. I know you'd love to skip the void. But that's where the magic is. Skip the void and sooner or later you'll find yourself back at the breakdown again.

So… the void. What do you do with it? You BE. You embrace it as if it is the greatest pleasure you've ever experienced. You invite it in for as long as it chooses to stay. You let go of all resistance. Soon after you give up the resistance, the void becomes addictive. The space. The pleasure. The joy. The ease. It's just one choice away. In its wake, it will leave you with new ways of going forward without your addiction to hard work, to stress, to being over-stimulated.

The void is the gift you give yourself when you need a circuit breaker with power to create true change.

BURNOUT
BREAKTHROUGH ACTION

How can you welcome the void? When the way forward isn't clear, be more and do less. Embracing the void allows you to receive its gifts. The void never arrives empty-handed.

> 1. Give yourself at least half a day a week that is just for you. It's amazing what no thinking and no talking can create. Begin to find pleasure in small things.

> 2. Go on a nurturing retreat where there is space to be you.

> 3. Sit in a dark room for a couple of hours with no other stimulation. Allow the space to nurture you. Allow whatever shows up to be there with no judgement.

Yes... it's the opposite of what you think you want. Trust me. I remember only wanting to do what I wanted to do. I didn't want a bar of the void. Now? It's my new drug of choice. It invites me into futures that I could not have imagined when my resistance was containing all possibilities and controlling all choices.

As you enter the void, your mojo begins to return. It loves the safe space of the void. It trusts the void, knowing it is the vessel that can liberate the real you.

INSPIRATION
& INSIGHTS

FINDING YOUR MOJO

Your mojo is your inner presence and an unstoppable energy of brilliance and being all that you are. That potency, zing, zest and flow that makes you know you're alive! That indescribable energy that sparks a magnetic attraction to all energies of bliss, making you feel like you are living in a superhero vortex of infinite possibilities. MOJO = MOre JOy!

When you combine this juicy, succulent energy of aliveness with a deep connection to your conscious awareness you create the magical energy of flow. No flow = no go!

Living through spaces of disengagement and disconnection from your inner essence is disconcerting at best and life-sapping at worst. A few hours or days can be manageable, but what to do when that tunnel of turmoil stretches far beyond what you ever imagined possible? How do you dig yourself out of that cavernous ravine of struggle, stress and stuckness?

Have you ever wished you could push a magic button so that your mojo would reappear instantly?

When Austin Powers famously lost his mojo he went on an outrageous adventure to rediscover his power, which of course was inside himself all along... Fat Bastard and Dr Evil could no more steal his mojo than fly to the moon... so everywhere you believe your mojo has been stolen or lost, would you be willing to give that up now and reclaim the brilliance of you? When your mojo flows, everything you touch grows.

PAUSE. BREATHE.

FLOW.

In his groundbreaking 1992 book 'Flow: The Psychology of Happiness' Mihaly Csikszentmihalyi described being in flow as "The state in which people are so involved in an activity that nothing else seems to matter; the experience itself is so enjoyable that people will do it even at great cost, for the sheer sake of doing it." For many, flow offers the experience of living beyond the limits of time.

His research focused on flow being experienced through activities that "provided a sense of discovery, a creative feeling of transporting the person into a new reality. It pushed the person to higher levels of performance, and led to previously undreamed-of states of consciousness."

The world has changed in extraordinary and unpredictable ways since 1992. We have become a lot more conscious and aware of possibilities in this physical reality and beyond. Imagine having this energy of flow and presence throughout all of your living, all of the time. Do you remember what that is like? Maybe you were about two the last time you had it?

The consciousness of flow now goes far beyond 'losing' our conscious self in activities. For me, flow is that space where whatever we play with comes to life with ease. Where the pieces of the puzzle fall effortlessly together. Where we just KNOW what else could be possible and that all is right with our world, even if logically it isn't! It is that space where we follow the energy of what we desire and it falls together with ease, instead of falling apart with dis-ease.

Are you ready to reclaim your inner bliss, get your giggle on and access that wellspring of joy that creates the energetic momentum you know and love? Or would you rather keep buying that old idea that nothing worthwhile can happen unless we suffer and struggle?

Living in flow is a state of BEing rather than DOing. It is being in the flow, and in the knowing of who we truly are. Life feels effortless. Workaholics, overachievers and highly sensitive people have a hard time allowing their flow to show up because they have spent so much of their life DOing so they could please others and prove their worth.

Is it time to stop suckering ourselves into that senseless struggle and stuckness that keeps us from being the magical mojo flow we truly be?

During my healing time, at the worst of the burnout, I cannot tell you how many times my acupuncturist tried to have me understand the essence of BEing. "What do you mean sit around and do nothing? Where's the joy in that?" was my invariable response.

BEing is simply foreign to us DOers. It has been an expansive and long journey for me in exploring the conundrum of BEing and DOing. I have discovered it is not about not DOing for the sake of doing, but about only taking inspired action, and then, when the magic shows up, there is a whole lot of joy in that. BEing does not literally mean doing nothing.

Being a high achiever or sensitive or an introvert... or investing our energy in upholding any personality traits we define ourselves by, are just ways of focusing our attention and our habits into a format that feels manageable and controllable.

What if we start with these traits (our current self-awareness) and choose a more conscious perception of what else is possible? If we are willing, these traits can transform into greater possibilities which may currently be outside of our imagination, and outside of the reality we have surrounded ourselves with so far.

As you read the next section... be kind to yourself. There's no need to judge yourself for what you haven't done or what you didn't know. You've already received way more than enough judgement! Living beyond burnout is about bringing new possibilities and choices to your awareness so that your life and body can show up differently.

I do sometimes wish I knew all this stuff when I was 20. What a different life I could have chosen. (You weren't thinking that at all were you?) Let's do a quick reframe before we start in on the juicy stuff.

One of my favourite mentors often says "You get it when you get it." It's never too late for you to choose the brilliance of you — whether you are 20 or 200! So, will you promise me you'll stop beating yourself up now? For what you didn't know because no-one told you? What if now is the perfect time? If you stop creating from the past, time literally won't be relevant!

BURNOUT BREAKTHROUGH ACTION:

Energise your life in one of these ways. Where will you start? If you haven't already, take the Amplify Your Energy Quiz (LivingBeyondBurnout.com/quiz) to discover what choices will make the greatest difference to you right now.

Change — not just your surface level habits... change the elements that will make the biggest difference.

Nurture — is not just symptomatic self-care... it's true nurture and nourishment of who you truly are.

Creativity — is not just about being an artist... it's about living creatively in every moment, through all of your choices.

Brilliance — is not academic or intelligence... it's embracing your super-powers and delivering them to the world in the ways that only you can.

If you're wondering 'how', the next sections will explore each of these elements in new and surprising ways!

INSPIRATION
& INSIGHTS

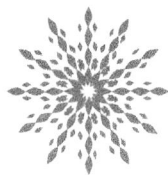

SECTION
II
THE BURNOUT
BREAKTHROUGH
MODEL

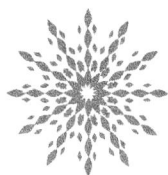

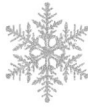

1. THE EASE OF CHANGE

CHANGE IS THE CATALYST

"It is we that make the choice, and the choice that makes us." (Sense8, Series 1)

Change has an undeservedly bad reputation. Most people think of change as an unwelcome imposition that is thrust upon them without choice. That kind of change often sucks. In contrast, the change that you choose, because you are seeking a greater future, is the kind of change that nurtures and expands your life.

You may imagine this chapter isn't for you. You're too tired and worn out or worn down to even consider changing anything. You just want to feel better. I thought that too. I took a month's leave from my job and all I wanted to do was sleep for the rest of my life. Sadly, even after a month of sleep and rest, I was not refreshed and revitalised. I was no closer to being well than when I started. That was the moment I knew that real change was required, rather than just band-aiding the symptoms. Change creates your future. Choosing no change recreates your past.

I have fought the burnout beastie a few too many times and I've come out the other side every single time – knowing more, being more and having greater awareness than I believed possible. If, today, you are sitting on the edge, going 'WTF?', I have written this for you. Sense it as a big energetic hug that can change everything in an instant.

The burnout beastie sneaks up on you, stealthily turning a once joyful life into a shattering string of moments of overwhelm and despair that sound like: 'Who am I and is this all there is? When will I get my life back?'

In the worst of those times, I remember hanging on by a thread, waking up every morning, wondering if the thread would hold another day. Wondering if it would be easier to just quietly, gently let go and allow the sad little burnout shell that was pretending to be me to just disappear into the nothingness... (which is not the same as the void!)

I remember not being able to keep myself upright for more than about 3 hours at a time and continually going back to bed and crying for no reason except total exhaustion. I remember not being able to remember the beginning of the sentence or what I was talking about, being so incoherent that I could barely answer basic 'yes or no' questions...

Questions like 'Would you like some chocolate?' were pretty much beyond my cognitive capacity to deal with (difficult to believe now I know!) It's a scary thing being 40 and seriously wondering if you have Alzheimers... For over 12 months my short term memory simply didn't exist. If I didn't write it down, I couldn't function.

It was clearly a less than ideal state in which to complete the MBA that I'd started when I still had my job. I am deeply grateful for my study buddies during this time. They were incredibly supportive and kind in the times that I couldn't keep it together. Funnily enough, it was during this time that I discovered how to use this capacity I have for being more than a little aware of other people's thoughts and all of the information that is floating around in space. There are many ways to do exams successfully... not all of them require rote learning! What if we could know what we need to know through awareness instead?

I remember being extremely unhappy because I couldn't live the life I knew was possible. It's been almost 9 years now since that was me. Most of all I remember wondering how in hell I had landed myself in such a mess and being terrified that it was never going to change. The burnout beastie had me so fried that

I couldn't decide if I should check-in to a psychiatric hospital or check-out... permanently. I am so grateful that my decision-making capacities were non-existent at that time. So grateful that I had disabled myself to such a degree that I literally had no capacity to choose anything except to just BE!

CHOOSING PERSONAL CHANGE

Despite my total incapacity, somewhere inside I knew that giving up could not create the different possibility I was truly desiring. I knew that whatever had gotten me into this mess in the first place had to change – massively.

What sticks us with burnout is that we always want the world outside to change. We want the world to conform to our aware-ness of what could be possible... and we want to take everyone we know with us... the burnout beastie shows up when we are doing so much to create change that we never just BE.

It was my addiction to creating change and generating greater possibilities in other people that wore me out and took me from being a catalyst for change, into a 'human doing' that desperately requires change. People who get burnout are never happy with the status quo. We know we have the potency to create a different reality and we want it now! It's how we go about it that sends us into the arms of the burnout beastie.

Imagining you are irreplaceable is one of the big lies that creates burnout. We tell ourselves a grand story about how much we care and how much we need to do to enable those around us to have different choices, mostly because they can't see what we can. That part could be true — they often can't — or maybe they just don't choose to?

I bought this big fat burnout beastie lie for a long time. How could things change if I wasn't there, driving it all forward? Always being the catalyst, always being there for other people, always making it easy for everyone… except the one person who needed it most… ME!

When the burnout beastie comes to visit, you can't be that for other people anymore… you don't have it in you! There is no steam left to power the train!! The party's over baby… you are officially on the intensive care 'do not disturb' list… until you change you… until you start caring for you… until you start feeding and nurturing the amazing being that is you. There is nothing for you to do except be. Yes. Change starts with the void!

Is it now time to put down all of the beasts of burden you are carrying around? Are you ready to look at what would truly work for YOU… and to actually just BE the possibilities you are aware of, rather than dragging the unwilling along for a bumpy ride down a dead-end track?

Yes, I know… you may have a whole lot of 'shoulds, have tos, must-dos' and 'oh buts' running around in your head right now. You can't possibly stop now — there are people relying on you — you need the money — life won't be worth living if you give up what you most desire to create.

Every excuse you can come up with I have tried… and tried… and tried… and what you need to know is that the burnout beastie is now driving the train — and he doesn't do train tracks! There are no refuelling stops, so you are on a collision course to nowhere — unless you change something fast.

PAUSE. BREATHE.
PLAY.

So this is what you are going to change. You are going to start sensing what you truly desire and you are going to start nurturing you first, before anything or anyone else. That's it. Turn off the phone. Cancel stuff. Change stuff… do whatever it takes to boot out the burnout beastie – it's time to refuel.

If you're not sure what refuelling looks like… here are three of my favourite ways to fill up your energy:

- Snuggle up with someone or something you adore…(even if it is a teddy bear or your dog!) …stop thinking… allow peace to infuse your universe and just BE. Let go of the guilt, the shame and the fear of collapse. It isn't going to help you heal.

- Laugh. Words cannot express how grateful I am for the friends who made me laugh and laugh and laugh until I stopped crying during the darkest of those burnout beastie days… they literally saved my life.

- Play. Oops… you've forgotten what that is like haven't you! Find a small child who has total delight in their world and rediscover a whole new universe of just being in the moment. Play is judged as a waste of time. What if it is the fuel that drives all possibilities? Seriousness is vastly over-rated.

I have a question for you: If you were choosing for YOU today, what would you choose?

Please know. If you are closer than you would like to the burnout beastie… this is not the end. It is the beginning of something greater than you have ever imagined possible, if you choose change now, rather than at the end of the track.

When I removed the burnout beastie from my life I lost the person I thought I had to be… and I became the person I could BE — the one that truly could change anything… just by BEING me… what if that could be possible for you too?

WHERE CAN YOU START?

What did I change first? I had to acknowledge that burnout was a way of slowing down or stopping the changes that would make my life more wonderful. On the surface it looked like there was far too much going on. In reality all of those things were skipping along on the surface. My being had much deeper and grander yearnings which were left unfulfilled.

In hindsight, I have realised that every single time I had burnout, there was an underlying need to make significant changes in my life. The burnout came because I hadn't listened to the quiet niggles of disquiet that an essential element to my happiness was missing; that I was out of sync with my true essence; that I wasn't being all I could be; that there was more to my life and work than was in front of me in that moment, even if I was pretending I was happy. Accomplishing more, being productive and having more money had failed to make me truly happy, even though I kept myself very busy doing those things.

Do any of these situations sound even remotely possibly like your life right now? Please don't panic. I'm not asking you to change it all today! I am asking you to consider if there is a scenario in your life or work that is literally tiring you out, wearing you down, even if it looks like winning lotto on the surface.

For example, you may have a dream job or dream partner that has a dark side that you haven't really acknowledged. You may be juggling a lot of projects you love, that aren't giving you quite as much love in return, leaving your well a little empty. You may be bored of your life, even though a lot of other people would be thrilled to swap places with you. It's time to be intensely honest with yourself. This is true kindness. Don't make yourself wrong, choose change! Do you know that you don't have to wait for something to be a problem to make a different choice?

BURNOUT
BREAKTHROUGH ACTION

Right now, ask yourself: "What change could I choose that would allow all burnout to dissipate?" You may have been instantly aware of what needs to change or your face may contort into its unabatedly mystified look. If you are instantly aware, now may be the time to write yourself an extremely personal love letter. Write about your gratitude for what your choice has created so far, and invite yourself to explore what change may be like in the new situation.

If you have been fanning the flames of burnout for a while, you may have no idea what needs to change because all of your limited energy is focused on managing the symptoms. It's also possible that the change that is seeking you is not yet definable - it's still evolving into what could be possible.

One way forward in these situations is to explore what could change by asking questions. These are questions that you don't know the answer to before you ask them. They may not even have obvious or immediate answers. Or you may have an instant 'aha' type response, your dreams may talk to you or the awareness may even come in conversations, at the movies or via a book. Carry a notebook or start a note in your phone to write down the inspiration you receive as you live your life.

QUESTIONS FOR GETTING CLEAR ON THE CHANGE YOU ARE SEEKING:

1. What would I like to upgrade?

2. What would I like to release or let go of?

3. What would I like to create in new ways?

4. What would I like to stop forcing?

5. What would I like to allow into reality?

None of these questions mean more work, more trying or more exertion. None of them are about perpetuating the past into your future. They are about acknowledging where you are and allowing the vice-like grip you have controlling your current situation to release and relax, so that you can begin to perceive the different possibilities that you could be choosing.

You may think that you can't leave your job or your partner (or your kids!). You may think you can't stop that side-project that you love more than anything. You may think you can't have an easier life in your current situation. You may think you can't add another thing to your world.

You may be correct, or you may not be. Until you begin to explore the alternatives, you won't know for sure what changes are available to you for moving forward. Don't resist the exploration, let curiosity be your guide in discovering what else is possible that you may never have considered. There are always multiple ways forward.

INSPIRATION
& INSIGHTS

ARE YOU TRYING TOO HARD?

One more thing. Is your perfection keeping you bound by burnout? Are you trying too hard? Working ridiculously hard to keep all the 'shoulds' in place? Stuck in a whirlpool of proving, perfection and peace-keeping? Exhausting yourself in the process? Stop it!

All try-hard behaviours are the result of incorrect assumptions. Are you trying to be something you don't think you are? Are you trying to be something you're not, because someone you care about thinks you 'should' change?

This is where perfectionism and over-work come from. A need to be 'more', without asking about the cost of trying. Trying sucks us dry and stops us from creating true change. When you remove trying from the situation, you can be present with what is, and what is actually possible, with a lot more ease.

What are three ways you try too hard to 'get it right'?

What three things are most exhausting for you right now?

We resist change when we think we have everything 'right' or when we think that what is coming will be worse or less than what we have right now. When you acknowledge the reality of your current situation, it opens the possibility for it to change. When you fight for your limitations or fight against change, the only person you make miserable is you. Is it time to ask yourself this: "What have you decided change is, that it actually isn't?"

Are you saying no to change? Or are you saying no to choice? Is there a change you are not making or asking for, just in case you lose what you already have? When you refuse change, you are saying you don't trust yourself. That lack of trust is a lack of knowing that you can make choices that will turn out greater than you can imagine.

PAUSE. BREATHE.

TRUST.

Let's play for a moment. Ask to be aware of the first choice that lead you into having burnout. As you made that choice, were you aware of a slight niggle, a heavy feeling, or a clunkiness around the choice? Did you listen to it or did you brush it off?

I'm willing to bet a lot of money that you had an awareness that this was not going to work out so well, even if, on the surface, everything appeared perfect. I've discovered I can usually track these niggles back to specific conversations, specific moments, specific creepy feelings that I ignored because I thought I knew better. Thinking yourself into or out of a situation really sucks if you are valuing it far more than your awareness. Trust your intuition rather than your mind. Your mind is sometimes a dirty liar, mostly because it doesn't have all of the information that your intuitive senses do.

To embrace change and allow it to create a new ease-filled future, start listening to the niggles and inklings in the moment they come to you and then have the courage to make choices that may on the surface seem crazy. Are you ready to stop doubting you and start trusting you? When you choose that, change will come with ease (and without burnout!!)

When you trust yourself, you know what you know. You perceive possibilities and make choices. You receive information and inspiration and know if it is relevant to you or not. You don't second guess yourself, don't doubt yourself and don't make yourself wrong for the choices you've made so far. What if everything is a contribution to your future? When you see that as a possibility, you will allow even the worst times of your life to create new ways forward.

One of the easiest ways forward is to have gratitude for where you are right now, even if it looks like a hopeless situation. Why? Because gratitude and judgement cannot co-exist. If you are judging your situation, you cannot change it. Being grateful for where you are (even if it is rock-bottom) is the start of creating new ways forward. Without gratitude, you'll continue to resist the small changes that snowball into bigger changes.

When looking at what you can change, it's too easy to get stuck in a treadmill of making yourself wrong for past choices. You can ask 'Why' and continue to create from the past, or you can ask 'What if...?' and create for your future. What if the greatest kindness you can be for you today is to stop making yourself wrong for 'not coping'... 'being too exhausted' ... 'being a failure' ... What if none of these judgements are true? What if having burnout is simply a dynamic course-correction device in action? Burnout is a pivot point, not an empty dry well.

After playing with the questions in this chapter, you may feel like an ant facing a mountain. Where do you start? You start by being present with the possibilities that are emerging. You aren't fixing what's broken, you're creating a greater and very different future.

"The secret of change is to focus all of your energy, not on fighting the old, but on building the new." — Socrates

BURNOUT
BREAKTHROUGH ACTION

If you have burnout, identify the top three changes that your life is asking of you. Which one of these changes can be most easily actioned? Identify one action you can take that will give you more energy right away and start there. Right now this is a step-by-step process, not a quantum leap into having so much change that you are so out of control that you end up shaking like jelly in the corner.

If you are supporting a friend or colleague with burnout, invite them to ask the questions in this chapter and explore new ways forward. What one change can you assist them to implement? Can you help them identify a couple of simple steps forward? Remember not to overwhelm them with either questions or choices. In the early stages of recovery, a gentle approach creates ease. One more thing. Please don't put words in their mouth! It is not for you to make choices for them, your job is to open up the conversation so that new choices naturally emerge. You are the catalyst, not the engine!

INSPIRATION
& INSIGHTS

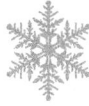

BEING PRESENT WITH POSSIBILITIES

"You can try to manage havoc, or you can nurture change."

Embracing the uncertainty of change means you must be present with the possibilities as they arise. Yes, I know it sounds scary. Your predictable reality no longer exists, but you're using an incredible amount of energy to keep it in place.

When you have burnout, it's tempting to check out, to go through the motions of change and being present without truly engaging. It seems like it is saving energy where in reality it is using more energy, as you miss the gifts and signals that would allow you to make a different choice. When you have little presence, your world contracts. When you increase how present you are, your world expands. Not into overwhelm. Into possibilities. Presence nurtures the expansion that change invites.

IS YOUR BREAKDOWN ACTUALLY YOUR BREAKTHROUGH?

This sounds counter-intuitive — how can a breakdown lead to a breakthrough? Not long after my third major meltdown I was blessed to have a short but insightful conversation with a wonderfully perceptive and gentle man about the meltdown merry-go-round I kept choosing.

I will never forget the moment this man asked me 'So what

is it about having meltdowns that is so rewarding for you?' The merry-go-round instantaneously stopped spinning. I knew what that energy was!! This was the aha moment I had searched for everywhere for more than 15 years and paid thousands and thousands of dollars for! When I was truly willing to know, the answer showed up, no charge. Here it is:

I create meltdowns when everything in my life needs to change.

Yes, every single time I had a big meltdown, I changed everything in my life. I turned my life inside out, upside down and forwards because, somewhere deep in my being, I knew I wasn't being true to myself. Did I have conscious awareness of this at the time? Absolutely not! Can I see it clearly now? Yes!

Where did that moment of total presence and vulnerability lead?

I am a lot more aware of who I truly be and what is required in my life for being me to be my priority. I am a lot more conscious of the times when I am not being true to me. I make incremental changes often, rather than allowing the meltdown momentum to burst into a crescendo of unlimited chaos. If I am heading towards chaos, I know there is something I need to look at and change — quickly!

Do I always get it right? No... still practicing!!! I still have the occasional mini-meltdown. I am still not totally aware of all of the moments and situations that take me away from BEing ME... but there's a lot less of them now and I know that the more conscious awareness I allow into my life, and the more I am willing to choose for me FIRST, the less these moments occur. It requires presence to choose for me. Without presence, I'm an automatic response system filling all the gaps in other people's worlds. Not so fun!

If how you are living feels like hard work you could ask yourself..."What am I trying to hold together that if it all fell apart would allow me to generate what I have never been willing to have or be?"

Have you ever been in a relationship that you just did not want to let go of, even though it felt like being dragged through a barbed wire fence backwards? When you finally let go, did you all of a sudden find you had the space, energy and possibility for things to be far greater and more blissful than they were? Did you find yourself falling into the flow of oneness instead? Often we hold relationships together instead of immersing ourselves in the oneness with the universe that makes everything possible.

What's infinitely amusing to me in situations like this is the insanity of our thinking. We believe holding on with a vice-like grip is what is keeping us together, but actually it has us stuck in the vice-like grip of a past that no longer exists! I remember the death throes of one relationship where we used to text each other 'I remember when....' stories as a way of trying to recapture the magic we had. Now I look at that and go 'was I crazy?' How much more ease could have been created so much sooner for both of us if we had been willing to let go of the stories from the past, be in the present and individually rediscover a new flow.

Anything you have a vice-like grip on keeps you from being in the moment. The reality is you have come to a conclusion about what 'should be'... Would you be willing to prise your fingers gently off whatever it is you are holding onto, wash them softly under some warm running water, shake them about a bit and get them all loosened up... and then let the flow take you to greater possibilities?

You can't be in the moment or see the moment for what it is while you have your steering wheel on full lock! Would you be willing to let go and create a totally different space for new possibilities to flow? When we are stuck in our fixed points of view and our conclusions about how it 'should be' there isn't a lot of room for the universe to create magic!

BEING PRESENT WITH YOUR BREAKDOWN CREATES YOUR BREAKTHROUGH

When I first discovered I was sensitive and in managing my energy consciously I could change everything in my life with ease, all I could think was 'Why?' 'Why didn't life give me an instruction manual at 15 instead of 40? Why didn't anyone ever tell me it was this easy to change? Why have I been struggling needlessly all this time?" On and on it went in my mind...

Until one day I woke up and decided to be grateful for my discoveries, and grateful that I have the gifts that allow me to share what I have learned with you! Why is not a question that takes you anywhere useful. In most cases it will take you into a victim-oriented spiral. Stopping the 'why' spiral was a true breakthrough moment — the past doesn't matter — it's what you do with the present moment that changes everything!

PAUSE. BREATHE.

BE GRATEFUL.

Wherever you are right now is perfect for you. Sure, you may wish to be somewhere else or in another body or brain that is not having the meltdown yours is!! All that means is that there is still the potential to choose a breakthrough instead of a breakdown. Let's explore how you can move forward.

A breakthrough can be characterised as a sudden, dramatic and important discovery, usually in relation to a perceived obstacle, which then allows for greater possibilities to show up. In simple terms, it's your 'aha' moment, when all becomes clear and the next steps appear with ease!

Breakthroughs come from understanding, new perspectives, connecting seemingly unconnected dots, being consciously aware, being creative, giving ourselves space, making mistakes, asking questions, trying out new choices, changing what's not working... Breakthroughs are everywhere if we are present with the possibilities, instead of focusing on the breakdown!

Before we can create breakthroughs it's sometimes easier to transform the stuck places that are stopping us from seeing the possibilities. Most non-sensitive people have the capacity to just leave that pile of crud on the ground and walk purposefully towards the new. As a non-sensitive friend of mine put it "Is there really that many people who need help with this stuff? What on earth would you talk to a therapist about?"

As acutely aware achievers, we are different. We feel the need to make all the piles neat and ordered, to sort out the shit and to make everything nice. It's a cute idea in theory, but it could have us wading through shit for the next 10,000 years. A lot of the new age, spiritual people want us to sort out every bit of rubbish before we move forward. I don't know about you, but I found that exceedingly tiresome. All that digging up of the past to find the tiny speck that wreaked the havoc is not a recipe for ease and joy!

The good news is we can move past the shit quickly and easily if we choose. Most of it can go straight to the bin, and there'll be a few gems worth redesigning. The bad news is a lot of us have the habit of wallowing in our garbage. So, you have a choice! Do you want to be baggage free or stinky?

If you are choosing baggage free, then being present and inviting presence will provide you with a space for clarity, so that your mojo returns and you can enjoy your flourishing flow once more! I can't help if you are choosing stinky!!

BEING PRESENT

This is the tool to use when all you can do is keep repeating 'I just have to get through today'. This mantra becomes a habit that makes every day just like the one before… not quite what you truly desire I suspect!!

There are times when we have so much happening in our business and our life that we almost forget to breathe! It is easy to revitalise your energy by simply becoming present in the moment.

Being present indicates you are acting in harmony with your environment, you are awake and you are acting with awareness of what you are creating.

Being present has three major advantages: firstly, you'll hear your intuitive awareness more clearly. Secondly, what you desire will come to you because you're actually here to receive it. Lastly, you'll escape from the pressures of overwhelm and overdrive as you will be living only in this moment — not in the hours, days, weeks or months ahead! Remember, your life happens in each moment — make the most of it.

In the moments when overwhelm threatens to send you over the edge, it can be very helpful to take just a few minutes to do something which will bring you back to awareness of the present moment… Here are my top five tools for becoming present right now.

- Breathe deeply for 10 — 15 breaths, do nothing except notice what is happening in your body — if it hurts anywhere, breathe into those spots to release the tension.

- Concentrate on slow meditative music to enjoy a rest from thinking. Tibetan singing bowls are very calming and easily available on YouTube... Or play music that makes you happy!

- Take a meandering walk around the block. Look out for butterflies, beautiful flowers and carefree smiles from small children... relax!

- Clear clutter. All that 'stuff' might still be there, but if it is not right in front of you it is much easier to focus on what's important... Visual people like to see their stuff. Discovering clear plastic folders has made my desk infinitely more organised!

- Immerse yourself in a relaxing warm bath using pure essential oils.

In coaching business owners, I often find that they have become so busy 'doing' that they are not living the idyllic life they originally set the business up to achieve.

If you desire to enjoy the benefits of living in the present moment, then fast does not always equal fabulous! I go through times when I am asking for everything to change faster... instead of it showing up faster, mostly I just become frustrated with the slowness. Not exactly a grand idea! When I immerse myself in the moment and have joy in what I'm creating, the speed seems to show up with ease. You cannot nurture or care for yourself or your ideas if you are not present. When you be totally present you have total choice.

WHEN YOU ARE PRESENT...

- You are aware of what is going on around you and in the world.

- You are 'with' your body.

- You are totally present with what you are creating, who you are talking with, what you are being, what is required of you...

- You know what choices and possibilities are available right now.

- You are aware of the future, and you can extrapolate with ease.

- You easily let go of everything that isn't relevant to now.

- You have clarity, ease, peace and a sense of everything being okay... no matter what is going on around you.

- You know you can't 'lose', whatever you choose.

- You aren't 'checked out', oblivious or distracted.

- You are being YOU, and you are connected with everything that is.

WHEN YOU HAVE PRESENCE...

- You have a clear, strong energy that is indefinable and yet unmissable.

- Your energy is 'visible' to people in the way you carry and conduct yourself.

- You are poised, unflappable, not controlled by others.

- You are a contribution to everyone around you — just by being YOU.

- You are always creating an invitation for people to choose more.

- You have a willingness for people to hear what you are saying.

- You don't judge, you are present with what is, which allows ease with change.

- You don't expect anything and you invite everything that is possible.

- You melt judgements and limitation by simply being.

- You have no point of view and you don't react to the points of view of others.

- You energetically own any room you walk into and any online group you are a member of... because your presence cannot be ignored.

When you are present and have presence, the crazy desire to control everything stops ruining your life. Control is having your foot on the brake and the accelerator at once...and it has the same effect. In essence you go nowhere but you rapidly burn-out your energy sources. What's better than control? Presence. It allows you to trust you at all times, no matter what is going on around you.

Having presence is a quality that few people are willing to master. Without presence there is always struggle. With struggle there is the lie of having no choice. Resistance to change is a resistance of choice. It is the unwillingness to choose the freedom that is available to you. Is this the life you truly desire to live? Or would you rather live a life that demonstrates your love for yourself and the world?

"When you love someone, the best thing you can offer is your presence. How can you love if you are not there?"
~ Thich Nhat Hanh

BURNOUT
BREAKTHROUGH ACTION

Being present is a muscle you build. You can start in any of these simple ways:

- Go outside. Listen to the symphony of the birds. Be aware of the sun or the rain on your skin.

- Be grateful for every tiny thing you can find. Not just the things you 'should' be grateful for.

- Choose anew in every ten seconds. Don't do anything by habit or rote. What choice is available to you NOW?

- Scrunch your toes a few times to bring your awareness into your body.

- Listen without judgement or conclusions. Don't form your response until the other person has finished speaking.

INSPIRATION
& INSIGHTS

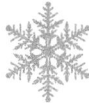

2. NURTURE & NOURISHMENT

NURTURE, NOURISHMENT OR SELF-CARE?

When I started getting noticeably unwell, well-meaning people advised me to rest more, give up my hobbies and study, to relax by doing as little as possible, to get massages, eat healthier food, exercise, meditate, connect with people I love and take more vitamins. This is the auto-pilot of self-care and it falls far short of what is truly required to restore yourself to the energised, alive, conscious being that right now may seem as distant as a minor character in a third-rate film that you saw twenty years ago.

In many cases, these are not the things that make the greatest difference to living beyond burnout. They are the surface level choices that keep your physical world humming along, but they don't provide the deep nurturing that your spirit is seeking. Nurturing, nourishing care goes far beyond the physical. It starts with knowing what feeds your joy at the deepest of levels.

I was horrified and confused when people suggested I give up on everything that made my life worth living to keep myself alive. When they suggested that I would have to live a slower, less active, less magical life. When they suggested I'd have to 'be careful' of my body for the rest of my life unless I wanted to end up in a wheelchair with chronic fatigue, fibromyalgia or some other life-sapping dis-ease. That was not living to me. That is what I knew as surviving. And it wasn't enough.

I was determined I would find another way forward... and I have. I now have more energy, more zest for living, more bliss, more creative possibilities, more of a sense of myself than I ever imagined possible before burnout. I've been travelling the world, speaking and running workshops. I live at the beach and I get to play every day. Even though I resisted the burnout like a child resists vegetables, ultimately it offered me a great gift once I started to embrace new and different possibilities. I had to be willing for my life to change, for it to be able to change. This was a huge hurdle initially.

I thought I had a great life. I did. A very limited great life. The life I have now is immeasurably more wonderful in just about every way. When you let go of what you imagine are the best choices you have, you begin to live and thrive in even more enjoyable ways.

THE DIFFERENCE BETWEEN SELF-CARE AND DEEP NURTURING

I discovered there is a world of difference between self-care and living a nurturing, nourished life that feeds the very essence of who you are. Self-care sits on the surface, like a tablecloth, protecting the you that you truly are from ever seeing the light of day. It's not that self-care is bad; it's just that if that's all you choose, it will never be enough. Not enough to create your recovery from burnout. Not enough to stop you from getting burned-out in the first place. Not enough to satisfy the calling of your brilliance or the expansion of your awareness. Not enough.

This is why most of the advice given about self-care and work-life balance falls short. It doesn't go far enough. Or deep enough. Or joyfully enough. Or playfully enough. Or gloriously enough. Or adventurously enough. It's the plain white tablecloth hiding a tired but dependable kitchen table, instead of offering a buffet of possibilities capable of creating lasting change.

A nurtured, nourishing life feeds you from the inside out. It is synergy in motion. It creates a multiplier effect where every choice you make has a ripple effect. When you live a nurturing, nourished life, your choices expand your possibilities for living rather than close them down. It includes your creative energies, your unique genius and your brilliance, and of course the physical activities that nourish your body and your being.

Self-care is too often about doing and it is mostly directed at your body. When self-care started being all about buying products and what someone else could do for your body, it stopped being the revolution that would invite people deeper into connection with who they truly are.

A lot of so-called self-care just becomes another thing on your never-ending to-do list. Self-care is the bandaid on a gaping wound that starts with judgement of who we are and what we are not doing, or what we 'should' do to be the powerhouse we tell ourselves we are. *Soothe your body with self-care, but don't expect self-care to cure.* For lasting change, you need to dive deeper.

If you have burnout or are always on the edge of a meltdown, I'd be surprised if you don't have a resistance to deeply caring for you. I hated the idea of self-care and all that nurturing stuff! It got in the way of my doing and helping and controlling and organising and being 'productive'! Oh the horror! I thought that was what I was brilliant at… little did I know. I was more than a little frustrated that all my doing didn't lead where I imagined it could. In hindsight, I'm hugely grateful. Those behaviours were all about the 'should'. The nurture and nourishment are all about creating a future where you are deeply, blissfully alive.

PAUSE. BREATHE.

BE KIND TO YOU.

Allowing yourself to create burnout is an unkindness to you. It's a way of perpetuating the suffering, rather than allowing a new, more authentic you to emerge. Are you being kind to everyone except you? Are those people receiving your kindness and being grateful for it? If not, you're putting a lot of your energy 'out there' with little return.

You can't flow energy in one direction only forever - to be fully energised and alive, you need plenty of energy flowing towards you. This is where kindness to you becomes a priority. Nurturing you starts with knowing you and adoring everything you are – even if you're not perfect! Especially if you're not perfect!

NURTURING YOU...

- doesn't mean you are lazy

- doesn't mean you are selfish

- doesn't mean you wait until last

- doesn't mean you must feel guilty

- doesn't mean you've failed

- doesn't mean you are needy.

If you were the most valuable energy in your life, how would you treat you? Do you treat your dog better than you? Do you treat your car better than you? What would it be like to be totally honouring of you?

STOP OVER-GIVING!

Are you living your life or everyone else's? It is common for over-achievers to have a big focus on helping others and doing for others. It's how we are trained and we spend our life forcing and struggling to get it all just right and perfect for everyone else in our life instead of living our own life.

We're taught that it is better to give than receive. Some of us have taken that far too literally! Look at the last three hours of your life. What percentage of your energy did you use in giving to others? What percentage of your energy did you use in giving to you? What percentage of your energy did you use in receiving?

A simple and powerful way to create intensive nourishment is to give yourself a minute or five between each activity. To not fill every moment with doing. To invite the space that allows you to receive the full energies of what you have just created or experienced. The pause offers awareness instead of busyness. When you pause, become aware of your body. Be grateful for it. Allow your mind to rest momentarily. Take a few deep breaths and gently move onto your next action. By becoming present with yourself in this way throughout your day, you start to acknowledge you. You're not a machine, you're a being that desires to be nourished.

BURNOUT
BREAKTHROUGH ACTION

How Can You Stop Over-Giving?

> 1. Ask for contribution from others, instead of being the one always giving.

> 2. Be aware of what you are aware of - just because you are aware of other people's needs, doesn't mean you have to act on them! Ask - "What will it create if I act on this awareness?"

> 3. Sit on your hands. Close your mouth. Stop being the first to volunteer. Allow others to contribute too!

When we choose to contribute to our own life first, this contributes to others. Would you rather be the perspiration or the inspiration? It is exhausting doing everything to make others happy, and its energising to be happy and inspire others by our example. Which are you choosing?

INSPIRATION
& INSIGHTS

PAUSE. BREATHE.

RECEIVE.

DO YOU LEAK ENERGY?

The weight of the undone will bring you undone. We leak energy in a thousand small ways. Unmet promises. Unfinished ideas. Unhappy conversations. Unawake choices. Unkempt environments. Unspoken resentments. Unchangeable routines. Unnerving worries. Unkind thoughts. Unclear targets…The undone is represented by all that is unloved in your life. Set your unloved free to be the true trustee of your energy.

As you begin to move beyond constant exhaustion, ask yourself what could create more nurture and nourishment. Here are a few ideas you can begin to explore once your physical energy emerges from its cage.

Unmasking you. Uncharacteristic adventures. Unraveled desires. Uncaged celebrations. Undoing the ties that bind. Untamed expression. Unabated enthusiasm. Unallocated time. Unfathomable joy. Unashamed curiosity. Unauthorised bliss. Unbiased discoveries. Unbelievable experiences. Unlimited connections.

You can see where this is leading right? Straight into unknown territories that will bring you alive. Now is not the time to resist. Persist in choosing something a little (or a lot!) different each day and the life you could be loving will unfold before your eyes. When you choose what will give you energy, rather than what takes energy, you come alive.

NURTURING & NOURISHING YOU

When was the last time you listened to you? Listened to what you truly desire for your life? Listened to what your life could be if you would just step off the treadmill for even an hour a day? Those first few tentative steps may feel strange. Slow. Suffocating. The different speed opens new doors. The different directions unleash new possibilities. It takes courage to get off the treadmill and see your life from new perspectives.

Start by rediscovering what brings you joy. By experimenting with what makes you feel playful. By breathing into the spaces that the dust of daily living has covered over. What have you given up that you used to love? What is ready for new ways forward? I know right now you may feel too tired to change anything, but if you're willing to ADD what makes you happy and let go of that which does not, you'll begin excavating misery and filling your well with joy.

Think of this time as dating yourself. You're about to get to know you in entirely new ways. I had no idea I love speaking in public, or that I was a writer, or that I could be happiest on days without any specific plans. I had no idea that I could paint, or that connecting with the earth would bring me so much pleasure. I had no idea that I was an angry cow and that underneath that was a strong, kind, potent woman. I had no idea that anxiety wasn't normal, until peace became my waking state. What is it about you that you have no idea about, that if you did, would turn your life into something extraordinary and phenomenal?

You thought you grew up when you were a teenager. Not exactly. Back then you learned all the 'shoulds' that were designed to keep you on the treadmill of what everyone on the outside wants from you. This time you'll grow up knowing who you are from the inside out. You get to be authentically you. When you be that, exhaustion falls away. It's tiring not being you!

You are looking for being outside of you, as if it can be fed on a spoon, inhaled, imbibed or infused. In truth, it cannot, although there are many spaces that invite the presence of being. In being, your life has more ease. You will not be looking for outside stimulation, or at what you are 'missing out' on - you cannot miss out. You can only enjoy being.

When you need to talk to no-one, it is so you can sense you, unadulterated, as it were - the purity of you. How often do you enjoy you? Or is this what is missing for you? Everyone except you gets to enjoy you.

BURNOUT
BREAKTHROUGH ACTION

Get a journal or notebook that makes you feel inspired. Take these seven questions and write about what they are to you, one a day each day of the week. Rinse and repeat for at least 4 - 6 weeks, without looking back at your previous insights until the end of that time. What's different? What did you discover? What have you changed?

1. What nurturing are you refusing to give yourself and what is the value of that?

2. If you are truly being you, who are you?

3. How do you express the true you in the world? How do you shut down the expression of you?

4. What is it about being playful and joyful that you most resist?

5. If you could choose anything, how would your life be a year from now?

6. What ease and harmony are you excluding from your daily life?

7. What are you making wrong about you or your situation that is actually right?

On the surface these questions may seem odd, irrelevant or not useful. I encourage you to be present with them. You might be surprised how the insights that come will allow you to make small but life-changing choices for nurturing and nourishing you.

INSPIRATION
& INSIGHTS

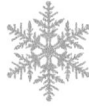

BEYOND THE BREAKDOWN

Stressed. Exhausted. Overwhelmed. Over-sensitive. Burnt-out. No contest, I was the CEO at Workaholics Anonymous for a long time... until I discovered that burnout comes when you've burned your energy supplies to below zero.

Before we get into the nitty gritty of energising you, there's something we must talk about. Something that rarely gets talked about. Something that needs airtime so that it is not a source of shame and embarrassment. Breakdowns.

I remember the first time I had a huge meltdown — I was 27 and everything in my life had collapsed at once — suddenly I had no job, no boyfriend, no joy. I had no idea what had happened to me, I chose to be born into a very practical family and I was brought up to 'just get on with it'. I had no context for how I felt, no idea of what to do with all the anxiety and overwhelm, no capacity to make sense of any of it, let alone get some help. So I ran away overseas, had three months off and came back thinking everything was normal.

Except it wasn't. The energy erosions that caused that situation were still simmering quietly under the surface. My core issue was I didn't know I was acutely aware and high-functioning autistic. I had no mechanisms for creating an energised flow for my particular type of wiring.

Being intelligent and sensitive has unique challenges. Intellectually you can deliver anything that is required, but energetically the delivery can be a rollercoaster unless you have a foundation of resilience and tools which allow you to operate consistently in a flow state. For many years I sat on the brink, always teetering between being in my potent flow, and having quiet (or not!) meltdowns where I wasn't coping with the intensity of what I was creating.

Breakdowns of any sort are rarely spoken about. Because I was always looking for 'the answer' to this challenge that kept coming back to haunt me, I was willing to talk about what had happened with many people. In so many conversations there would come a point where the person would say to me 'I've never really told anyone this, but do you remember when I had the 'xyz' job and all that stuff happened? Well I had a bit of a breakdown around then...' And so their story would be shared... and in sharing their secret, the feelings of shame, fear and embarrassment would start to dissipate.

There is nothing wrong with having a breakdown, whether it be physical, mental or emotional – it's just not that much fun!!

Breakdowns are a catalyst for change - nothing more, nothing less. Making them wrong makes change wrong. Without change, there is no evolution into greater futures. Whether they are personal or planetary, breakdowns have the purpose of creating change.

In being willing to be vulnerable about my idiosyncrasies I discovered that many people experienced what I had, in their own individual ways. It is time to stop the cover-up. The ways we have been living and working do not work for so many people! Our systems and structures are built to be hard on people, maybe not deliberately, but that is the effect of seeking profit and power rather than valuing people.

Please be aware that if you have had a breakdown (or are having one right now) then you are definitely not alone. My informal conversations with hundreds of people over the years would indicate you are closer to the majority than you realise!! It's likely that many people you know have had meltdowns. While in that space they did not know if or how they would ever truly recover.

If you are a leader, or simply a caring co-worker, look around you and see the beautiful amazing people who are currently at risk... and start to care — for you and for them. Together we create a different future.

PAUSE. BREATHE.
CONNECT.

If your health and wellbeing only become important when you don't have them, start to notice where you are nurturing and nourishing you and where you are being mean to your body. Disease is actually dis-ease. If your health isn't a priority your body will let you know that change is needed so that you can thrive and allow your life to flow.

You are a human BEing, not a human DOing. The essence of you is BEing YOU, not what you do!! Irrespective of what your inner critic or your external boss says, the only thing that will really make a difference in your life is BEing YOU…

In finally breaking through my own resistance to caring for myself, I have come to know that contrary to our conditioning and the 'perform or else' cultures evident in many workplaces, there is absolutely nothing in life or in business that is ever worth having a breakdown over. Not relationships, not jobs, not money, not health, not anything!!! All these things we make so huge in our mind will rarely matter next year, let alone in five or ten years. And yet, we continue to create situations that take us to breakdown.

What else is possible here? What if we looked at our breakdowns as the key to our breakthroughs? (That doesn't mean you need to create a breakdown every time you want a breakthrough!!) Could this different perspective on breakdowns create greater possibilities than we can currently imagine?

WORK-LIFE BALANCE? OR BLISS?

Work-life balance must be one of the most over-used and misunderstood ideas the gurus have come up with in the last hundred years! Let's take a look at what balance is really about. But first some clarifying semantics… you know the 'work-life' bit? Well that's included and there's a whole lot more to this too… so let's just call it balance!

BALANCE IS NOT…

Giving equal time to everything in your life — impossible and the fastest way known to adding to your stress!

An either/or universe — for example, a choice between having success or changing the world - in most cases you can do everything you desire, with a few new perspectives added to the mix!

BALANCE IS...

Having full awareness of what will create ease and joy — across all areas of your life.

Nurturing you first - when the well is dry no-one can drink from it, including you.

Investing your time in energising the harmony between you, your relationships, projects and interests.

The manic buzz around balance turned it into just another impossibly exhausting dream to strive for, mostly because the definition of balance assumed equality rather than harmony. Years of seeking balance only made me miserable. In trying to give equal love to everything and everyone, there was always some part of my life that felt 'missed out', because it just wasn't possible. Seeking balance became another exhausting 'to-do', rather than a choice for bliss!

I realised seeking balance was not enough for me. My real desire was to 'have it all', without having to compromise. Say what??? I know... it seems slightly ridiculous, and yet, it is brilliantly correct.

My idea of 'having it all' is having everything that thrills me, in whatever ways are possible, in the moment I'm in. I'm not talking about having a perfect life or being superwoman. My idea of 'having it all' is a moment by moment choice to be present, to live joyfully and lead boldly. That's bliss!

PAUSE. BREATHE.

CHOOSE EASE.

WILL YOU CHOOSE EASE?

Having it all starts with the choice to have ease. Do you resist ease as if it is a deathly disease? As if having ease will make you less important, less driven, less valuable? No... it allows you to create bigger, bolder and be able to offer even more value to the world — at less cost to you.

The real disease of balance is a wicked addiction to the cult of busy — doing all the 'shoulds' without question, and meeting all the expectations others have of you. If you're seeking a more delicious life full of everything you adore, leave the party of busy, via the door that says EASE!

If you only have to choose ease in each moment, you create life on your terms, rather than staring with big overwhelmed bug-eyes every time you catch sight of your to-do list.

HOW DO YOU START CHOOSING EASE?

1. Your glorious, magical ease-party starts with how you do the small things.

When we're busy, we imagine the small things don't matter. They do. But not for the reasons you think! (And definitely not because you 'should' do them!)

Small choices lead to big choices. When you create your small choices in nurturing, ease-filled ways, you train yourself to allow your big choices to show up like that too. Bigger doesn't have to mean harder, longer or busier when you know what choosing ease is like.

What do I mean? Is your kitchen set up to make breakfast quickly and easily? Do you have simple systems for the basic activities in your life? These are small choices that make a big difference to your energy levels. Bigger choices begin when you create what gives you pleasure, rather than what you imagine will deliver the perfect life.

2. Ease creates momentum.

The only reason we seek balance is because we can't fit everything in. We think the problem is time. It's not. Momentum out-creates time, every time!

Momentum has a creative flow that keeps everything moving forward. You begin to create outside of time, rather than containing everything into manageable time-slots that make you feel like you live in a prison of your own making. Flow is a continuing breakthrough where your priorities effortlessly evolve.

You know the story of pulling out one thread and the rest unravels with ease. Life is like that too! Ease is just a thread you pull, rather than a knot of threads you spend hours untangling before you can even start. Ask yourself..."What is the easiest way forward for me right now?" Start there!

3. Your energy determines your ease.

What energy do you create with? Struggle? Or ease? Making everything hard, or constantly fixing problems, so you can prove how fabulous you are, is not how to have it all. That is your addiction to approval shouting at you. You can listen to it, or you can say goodbye to all the ways you make your life harder than it needs to be.

Your crazy life can nurture and energise you when you start asking 'How can this be easier than I imagine possible?' The question opens up possibilities for new ways forward - you don't need a ten step plan. Start by inviting ease and allowing it space to do its magic when it arrives.

In the beginning your new choices for ease and flow may seem subtle, or small. Choose them anyway. Ease is a snowball and you are on the downhill run. It's time to stop pushing shit uphill in your quest for balance. There are no rewards for struggling with balance. Instead, you can celebrate the ease of living... your way.

Having balance comes from continual fine-tuning rather than trying to have perfect balance at all times. Think of it like riding a bike or rollerskating. Different directions require different momentum. You will dip in and out of success. If you are in the flow most of the time you will have a successful life. Remain awake, alive and aware so you can adjust in each moment.

BURNOUT
BREAKTHROUGH ACTION

Ask questions about every choice you have! Will you choose ease and energy? Or balance and burnout?

· Be in the moment —"What's next?' is a great intuitive question that will bring flow to your day if you are willing to stop forcing outcomes based on everyone else's expectations and points of view.

· 'Who could help me with this?' is another favourite. Go with the first person that comes to mind and call them. I've discovered that the world is full of people who will help you, if only you are willing to ask! Asking does not constitute failure.

· 'What would this be like if it was ease and joy?' will help you look at a situation and perceive it differently. Follow up with 'What would it take to change this?' and you'll be on your way to new and bliss-filled possibilities!

· 'How much fun can I have here?' is a stunningly simple way to take yourself less seriously. Remove the intensity of the pressure cooker and adjust your world using the elements of fun, play and laughter.

INSPIRATION
& INSIGHTS

BECOMING SELF-ENERGISING

There is a tendency to see our energy levels as something out-side of us, as beyond our control — "I wake up tired" "This is exhausting"... rather than questioning what choices would give us more energy in each moment. There is another perspective that says do more (exercise) to have more energy. When I had burnout the third time, I was encouraged to sign up to a personal training program which instantly sent my energy levels spiral-ling backwards. At that point, taking my body to bootcamp was a cruel and useless approach. Forcing your body to perform when it needs nurturing care and deep nourishment is crazy.

At the same time, some activities were giving me energy. Laughing with friends, playing with my cocker spaniel, planning my house renovations all filled the well. If you have guilty tendencies it's tempting to stop these kind of things too, as if it's wrong to have any kind of pleasure when you can't fulfil your obligations. No, it's wrong to make your life or work so miserable that you can't fulfil your obligations. (I won't get started on the topic of obligations here, or this book will turn into an encyclopaedia. Suffice to observe that so often obligations are 99% in our imagination, or based on other people's expectations, rather than a reality. There is no choice in feeling obliged.)

You know it's time to begin a self-energising adventure when you have energy for scrolling through Facebook from your pool lounger, but not enough energy to go move your body or meet-up with someone interesting... When you have energy to clean your office, but not enough energy to write something world-chang-ing... When you have energy to do the work you 'have-to' but never quite create what inspires you... When you have energy to show up in small ways, but you won't allow your true brilliance to be seen... When you have energy to (fill in the blank with your tiny choice), but not enough energy to (fill in the blank with your big choice). Does any of this sound familiar?

Energy emerges from the tiniest choices towards pleasure, possibilities and play. These choices are life-giving and choice by choice, your energy will begin to emerge. When it does, don't repeat the patterns of your past. Don't heave yourself straight back into working like a slave. Don't give that precious energy to the first person who demands it of you. Nurture it. Enjoy it. Luxuriate in it.

This is going to be uncomfortable. You'll resist it. And there will come this magical moment where you realise that you are at last using your energy for you, rather than against you. If you aren't willing to enjoy the energy available to you, you start using your energy against yourself. It feels like one step forward, two steps back because it is... if you aren't putting you first.

When you are self-energising, you won't diminish your energy for other people or situations. What are you tired of? Dig a little deeper than 'tired of being tired'. Are you tired of being less than who you truly are? Making less of an impact? Are you tired of the demands on you, so you allow the tired spiral to circle downwards so that those requests will go away?

PAUSE. BREATHE.

ENERGISE.

Another possibility is that you are you keeping a lid on your energy so other people can be happy. How much energy are you using to stop being as energised as you could be? If you are always modulating your energy for other people's ease and comfort, it's exhausting and unkind to you. If you want to sleep all the time, stop adapting you for other's expectations. What is the greatest expression of your energy in this moment? If you weren't diminishing your choices, your ways of being in the world for the comfort of others, how much energy would you have? When you explore this side of self-energising you invite resilience to take a seat along side you.

Being self-energising includes resilience, but not as you know it! Resilience doesn't ask more of you; it asks you to receive what you have, and be who you truly are. Have you misidentified what resilience actually is?

- It is not working beyond the point of exhaustion.

- It is not your capacity to bounce back by putting on a fake happy face in the face of non-stop obstacles.

- It is not putting yourself last or suffering for your work because you can't see another way forward.

- It is not your willingness to soldier on and bear the brunt of the fall-out around you.

- It is not your ability to keep producing and delivering, even if you have nothing left in the tank.

- It is not saying yes to back-to-back meetings or an unreasonable workload 'because you can' or because you imagine that other people expect you to.

- It is not about toughening up so you can do more.

- It is not about doing even more to please others or meet your quotas or targets.

Resilience is your capacity to recharge your energy. It's your choice to be well-restored. If you don't choose beyond constant busyness, you'll always be facing the scenarios above.

How do you recharge your energy? Not the way that you've been taught by the schedules that society expects of you (even though you think that's the answer!)

Wake up, go to work, work hard, endure the commute home, look after your family, fall into bed exhausted... do it all again tomorrow. It's what most people call living, but this is not living! It's surviving until your next day off. Sound familiar?

Do you treat your energy like most people treat religion? You'll have a rest once a week and during holidays (at best!), but you won't allow yourself to be energised by a deep and nurturing way of living? Is it working for you? I guess not if you are reading this book!

Your capacity to recharge needs to be available 24/7, not just occasionally 'when you have time'. What does that mean? Building recharge space into your daily life. Not as another scheduled 'thing to do', but as a way of living moment by moment, choice by choice.

Recharging is much simpler than we imagine. It is allowing small spaces in between the busy to be used for our enjoyment, rather than used against us by diving into the next thing without even a breath!

What's my secret to instant recharging? Being 100% present in what you are doing. Immersion, not diversion! Allowing the spaces in-between to be space rather than filling every moment with stimulation and being on the go. Living is being; busyness is the slowest, most painful death you can choose. What would it be like to treat your body as the gift it is?

BURNOUT
BREAKTHROUGH ACTION

How much energy do you have right now?

-1 I'm so exhausted I can't even read this.

1 I remember having energy once... about 5 years ago.

2 Energy? Isn't having no energy 'normal'?

3 I'm erratically energetic. Or maybe just erratic!

4 I have enough energy for what I have to do, but I'm SO bored, uninterested or tired.

5 I'm energised and alive... and sometimes I stop myself from being 'too much'.

5+ Energy? I'm dangerous! What do I do with all this energy?

Go to www.LivingBeyondBurnout.com/EYgift to receive your free *Energise YOU* guide. It's full of inspiring questions to move you beyond the energy level you're stuck at right now.

INSPIRATION
& INSIGHTS

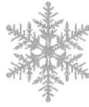

YOUR BODY IS A GIFT,
NOT AN OBSTACLE!

I know… right now you might hate your body. You're mad that it's let you down. You're frustrated that you can't seem to fix it with a couple of days off, a binge-drink, yoga or some vitamins. You hate that you are tired and fatigued 99% of the time. You are miserable even when you do have time off because your body isn't up for doing much of anything at all. You possibly want to cry at just about everything and you're wondering where happy, fit, playful, joyful YOU has gone. (That you will come back when you give your body big love, I promise!)

I remember that phase. And I remember how all that angst stopped me from being aware that the 'limitations' and 'obstacles' my body was displaying at every turn were just my body trying to help me get back on track. My body wasn't being difficult. It was trying to help me. At the time, I didn't see that and I was compounding the issue by fighting my body. So that you don't have to go down that long and winding path to nowhere, here's what I know now.

Your body is wise, so wise. And it's gentle too. It's been giving you subtle hints for years now. But you didn't listen. Please don't make yourself wrong. Please stop judging you and your body. Please start listening to your body. Please start having gratitude for your body. This is the start of not only recovery, but having more energy for living than you imagine possible right now!

Your body isn't the problem. It is giving you symptoms so that you'll make changes. Don't shoot the messenger! Your body operates like the cat's whiskers or the canary in the coal-mine. It has these extremely subtle sensing mechanisms that tell you almost everything you need to know about your life. And when you repeatedly ignore the tiny hints it gives you to keep you on track, it gets louder and louder and louder, until it has to scream at you with non-stop aches, pains, miseries and exhaustion. Do you think your body is happy about this? NO!!!! It doesn't like suffering either. But it is willing to do this so that you can both be a whole lot happier!

When I was judging my body for everything it couldn't be and do, it could only give me more of that. When I started being grateful for my body, the energies of tiredness and fatigue began to shift into new spaces of possibility and my energy started coming back. When I became over-excited and used that fresh energy to create more of the same (i.e. overwork and over-giving) my body would become fatigued almost instantly. When I used that energy to begin to create a new and very different life, I would receive more energy to expand into the possibilities. (Creating a different life is a big topic... we explore it deeply in the *Amplify Your Energy Lounge* weekly conversations.)

The world will not fall apart without you! In fact, if you have burnout, it is not you keeping the world together, it is the world that is keeping you together. What???

Your body was made for bliss, not burnout. It loves play, nature, movement, deliciousness, sex, adventures, expression, touch, nurturing the senses and space. It doesn't love working non-stop, being attached to a screen 24/7, being ignored, being forced to perform or being mistreated with food, chemicals, alcohol or violence.

WHERE CAN YOU START?

Experiencing pleasure and joy in your body is the beginning of a more expansive energy that can generate bliss throughout your life.

Know what makes your body feel good! The smell of freshly cut grass, ocean breezes, sunshine, the luscious juiciness of a slice of cold watermelon in summer. The feel of your bare feet on the earth. The beauty of someone massaging your feet. Wearing comfortable shoes and walking outside at lunch time. Eating just enough to satiate your hunger, rather than stuffing yourself so full that your body has no energy for anything except digesting food.

If your body is sending you noisy signals that it's time for change, asking your body a question like this "Hey body, what can we choose today that will allow this to change?" begins to invite new choices. And then do or be whatever pops in your awareness. Please honour you and your body by following through, even if the requests are weird or strange. If your body is asking for sweet potato toast, it knows that is what will nurture it the most right now. If it asks to sit or lie in the sun, enjoy it! If it asks to not work hard (i.e. to work easy…), or to have a mostly people free day, then find a way to choose that too.

Your body knows. When you listen, it can change. Fixing the symptoms will only ever be temporary. Learning to listen to your body's requests is the gold you've been paying therapists to create for you. They can't. When you listen, acknowledge and take the actions your body is asking for, it will create more energy than you know what to do with!

You probably think this is too simple. If you're used to doing everything from your head, this strategy won't be nearly complicated enough to change anything… or will it? It sounds easy. You have nothing to lose and everything to gain. So explore it for a day or a week and notice what changes. At first the changes will be subtle. You may not even notice them. If you keep going, you'll wake up to discover that you have so much more energy than you had a few weeks ago.

How Does Simple Self-Care Nurture Your Body?

You hoped I wouldn't mention self-care didn't you. Because that is the thing that is either last on the list or not even rating a mention. If you get a massage once a month or walk to the letterbox you think your self-care needs are satisfied. Not exactly!!

I resisted the basics of self-care like crazy too. And this is what I noticed. When I have clean sheets, all my clothes washed and put away, clean, tidy living spaces and nurturing, healthy snack food available, it is the start of having ease. With ease comes a sense of peace. With peace comes the ability to listen to my body even more closely. It's all interconnected. You can start with whichever choice works for you.

Notice I didn't put weekly pedicures and massages on that list of basics? That's because they are nice to have, but not essential when you don't have the basics in order. If you need to, get a cleaner or a friend to help you get the basics in order. When I first quit my job, my mum came to visit every day for the first couple of weeks (thanks Mum!!). She knew I didn't have it together enough to sort out even the basics. She helped me do things and she gently showed me how to put things in order (still not exactly my strong point... but I do at least have a place for everything now!)

Also, be aware that every time you resist basic self-care, you use up energy that could otherwise be nurturing your body into a happier space. Fighting yourself takes so much more energy than choosing to get dressed, choosing to eat a simple fresh meal, choosing to sit in the sun for ten minutes. Start with what you can, even if it feels like it will take the next ten thousand years to make any progress. You will surprise yourself when you stop fighting you!

The question is, are you willing to have ease with your body, or would you rather keep your limiting beliefs about the importance of struggle, stress and stuckness?

We can buy our own story, make it significant and use it as an excuse for everything that is not flowing in our living, or we can keep moving forward into the flow by asking for nurturing, nourishing, joyful energies to flow into all that we be and do. It is that easy. When we ask, the universe delivers.

PAUSE. BREATHE.
LISTEN.

LISTENING TO YOUR BODY

I used to be a walking, talking head. I ignored my body almost totally. It was a nuisance. Something that got in the way of what I desired to create. After the third round of burnout in 15 years, I had to acknowledge that my body not only existed, but that it had its own brilliance. It knew I couldn't stay in those jobs and relationships that weren't working for me, even though I pretended to myself that they were.

It took a while, but I finally realised that my body is way smarter than me. It is willing to know the things I am sticking my head in the sand about. It was willing to create a different reality even when I was doing my best to stay stuck in the linearity and logic of this reality. And I'm beyond grateful.

A whole new world opened up for me when I began to ask my body 'Hey body, what do you know about this?' Below are just a few questions you could ask your body so that you can start creating your future together, instead of as adversaries.

And when you ask these questions, listen to your body, not the people who are telling you what is 'good' for your body! What do I mean? Well, every time I travel internationally, I ask my body how it can re-energise the fastest and with the most ease. Sometimes it desires energetic bodywork, or a day or two at the beach, and sometimes it simply desires sleep — 24 hours of it!

On one trip, it asked for at least 24 hours off the internet and the computer! I don't have any point of view about how we connect with being in Australian time again - and I don't make my body suffer along the way. I leave space in my schedule for whatever my body asks for. Most people say you get over jetlag by 'staying awake until it's bedtime, no matter what it takes.' What if that is the least kind way of allowing your body to adjust its energy levels?

Just for fun, hug your body… show it that you adore it as much as it adores you. And know that it is not permanently broken — your choices can allow it to be an even more wonderful body than you had before burnout!

Burnout is not a life-sentence where your body does the punishing. It's an invitation to create a greater life than you've ever had before. Will you say yes to the party of your life? Or will you keep your outsider status, always looking for the quick fix, but never finding lasting happiness.

In most cases, our bodies need far less food than we give them. We use food as a sedative that slows us down. A lot of energy is used in digesting food. When I'm tired, I make my meals liquid. It gives me far more energy!

Please know, I'm definitely not suggesting you become a breatharian, or that you eat less than you need. I'm asking you to tap into what your body is truly asking for, so that it can show you how to have more energy. If you have adrenal fatigue, it's also useful to look at small snacks that support your adrenal functioning with more ease. Anthony William (the medical medium) has excellent resources on his blog for supporting your adrenals through food.

BURNOUT
BREAKTHROUGH ACTIONS

Here are the questions for having a deep and dynamic conversation with your beautiful body... (and feel free to create your own!)

· Hey body, what would give you energy today?

· Hey body, would you like to move today? If so how?

· Hey body, is there anything that would allow you to move beyond this burnout with more ease? Can you show me exactly what or who can contribute?

· Hey body, what kind of rest would be most generative for you right now?

· Hey body, what do you know about this that I'm not willing to know?

· Hey body, are you tired, or are you relaxed? (It's so easy to mix these two up!)

· Hey body, is it alcohol or something else you desire? (Are you drinking too much for your body to handle?)

· Hey body, how much food do you desire? Can you tell me when you've had enough?

INSPIRATION
& INSIGHTS

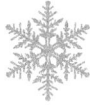

3. CREATIVE ENERGIES

DISCOVER YOUR
CREATIVE POWER

"Be regular and orderly in your life, so that you may be violent and original in your work." – Gustave Flaubert

Do you wake up miserable? Uninspired? Wishing you were going anywhere except to work? Or not wanting to get out of bed even if it's the weekend? This is the moment where you can choose to inspire yourself rather than fall into a slump. To inspire is to 'breathe life into', or to be 'influenced by the divine'.

This is what I discovered... When nothing interests you and you can't muster the energy for anything, it is your spirit crying out for nourishment. You the being cannot thrive when your creative energies are ignored or squashed.

If you don't think you're creative (or you're just too tired to be creative) it will be tempting to skip this chapter. Please don't. Your creative energies are not just about artistic pursuits. They are the essence of you. They feed your sexual energies, your sense of aliveness, and the expression of your spirit. When your creative energies are vibrantly alive, your creative power is in full flow.

When your creative energies are deadened or divided, it feels like the death of who you truly are. When I made the mistake of moving in with a narcissistic boyfriend, he tried to physically and energetically give me no space to be creative (or to be me). By this time, I knew the value of my creative energies and there was no way I was allowing that. I found a wall that was all mine and it became a beautiful expression of me through a friend's marvellous suggestion to create Soul Collage® cards. I found a photograph of that wall just recently and I was amazed at the power and potency in those images. I knew exactly who I was, even in the midst of abuse disguised as love. I just wasn't living it during that relationship!

Is there a creative expression of YOU that is suppressed? Or acknowledged but not being lived? Or even hiding? What simple action can you take to open up an authentic expression of who you truly are? Creativity saved my life... and now it energises my life.

PAUSE. BREATHE.

BE OPEN.

Are you excited to discover what's possible here? Or are you freaking out about how bad you were at art? Creativity isn't about art, it's about the expression of you and your ideas.

WHY BE CREATIVE?

- It makes you happy.

- It relaxes your body.

- It expresses the essence of your energy.

- It allows your business or work to grow and expand with ease.

- It invites new choices and possibilities that make sure you can never be bored.

- It shows you the way forward when planning is going nowhere.

- It allows the quirky expression of ideas.

- It stops you from getting burnout.

- It showcases your brilliance in ways that cut through the clutter.

In my book '*Stop Waiting, Start Creating*', I explore the topic of creativity in far more depth. For now, just know that every single person on this planet has unique ways of being creative. Your way may be totally different to your partner, BFF, or the people on your team. There is no right or wrong and it's not complicated. Creativity is simply about creating something different or new. It can take any form and use any materials or energies.

What do you know about being creative that you've not been willing to acknowledge? When was the last time you were creative? What is stopping you from being creative now?

CREATIVE UNSTICKING

All this talk about creativity sounds wonderful, but what if you're stuck creatively? Creative blocks can be frustrating. You are willing to do the work, but the inspiration just isn't there. While you wait for brilliant ideas to finally arrive, you may be burned out, frozen over, wading through mud or feeling blanker than the air we breathe! Start by playing with the element that flows... Water can create flow where nothing else will.

During my stickiest, stuckiest moments, a visit to the beach inevitably allows stuck energies to roll away with the outgoing tide. The hang gliders float in the breeze, the surfers are being one with the waves, the standup paddlers balance the ebb and flow and little ones squeal with delight as inflowing waves break over them, washing away sand castles and delivering new experiences. Immersing myself in this reminds me of the infinite layers of flow and joy available if we will just go with the energies that are present right now, in this moment.

Water is like a sneaky ninja. It can go places and make massive impact without a trace. It can seep through the tiniest of spaces and fill the entire sky in seconds. Where can you discover the tiniest trickle, the easiest path, the smallest stream that will open the floodgates to creative flow once again? Start there, in that tiny place and allow yourself to feel the full joy of the moment. What can you perceive? What can you receive right now? A glimpse of an idea? A word? A colour? A longing to explore a topic that could just have the potential of leading you to a real 'aha' moment?

Walking along the beach I breathe in the squeals of joy, the bliss of the bodies as they soak up sunshine, squidgy sand beneath their toes and luxuriate in the seductive salt air. I breathe in the ocean of possibilities and I play with all of the luscious energies that have contributed to the magic of this day. And when I create... and it flows with so much more ease!

Do you have great ideas in the shower? Maybe it's because we wash off all the outer layers of 'stuff' from our day or our dreams, and we literally step into the flow! It is a form of moving meditation – the physical actions don't require thinking, so we go easily into a flow state. Or maybe it's because we are alone and have time to reflect, without judgment, analysis, deliverables or expectations.

How can you play with water right now? If you are stuck in an office and nowhere near water, you can play with this energy immersion tool to bring water into presence for you. Immerse yourself in these moments of play...

BURNOUT
BREAKTHROUGH ACTION

(Find the audio of these playful energy immersions at www.LivingBeyondBurnout.com/inspire)

Ten Seconds of Play:

Imagine it raining possibilities into all the catchment areas of your life. Watch the waterfalls, creeks and rivers pour these possibilities into the oceans of abundance that surround you, see storms clearing out all the old energy that has you stuck... and then watch the flood of possibilities come streaming into your consciousness!

Ten Minutes of Play:

Connect with the energy of the ocean, being aware of every droplet being a new possibility that you could choose. Run your hands through the bubbling water... what will you choose? Watch the waves recede, what gifts do they leave behind? Take yourself further out beyond the breakers. Dive deep, feeling that cold wave of pure cleansing water wash through you. Look through the depths to see what treasures are there for you and know that when you resurface you will be refreshed and full of clarity.

Now take a beautiful boat across to a distant island, in the peace, calm and serenity, breathe deeply and recall exactly what you are creating. See how your recently discovered gifts and treasures contribute to the flow of all that you are. Be in total flow as you lie back and relax on this gorgeous island. Everything you require is here. You can stay as long as you desire. You don't need to go anywhere else, be anyone else or know anything else except for everything that is in your awareness right now. You are one with the All That Is. You have everything you can imagine and then some!!

When you are ready, the tide will turn. You can gather up your gifts, treasures and insights and place them safely in your awareness. Place yourself in the boat and it will gently float you back to shore... no effort required, it knows exactly where to land you for your highest wellbeing. When you arrive you will be exactly where you need to be, with the most awesome people who will contribute to your vision, and you will be immersed in the flow energy that will generate total ease and joy whatever you choose. Take a deep breath and know that everything is going to be greater than it has been before.

INSPIRATION & INSIGHTS

DREAMS, FANTASIES & POSSIBILITIES

Dreams do come true. Fantasies are an entertaining escape from reality. Possibilities are choices that are both available and able to be actualised. If you seek to be productive in your creative flow, it's useful to know the difference!!

Dreamers are people who know that a different possibility is available. Dreams come true if you have no point of view about what you are creating. "It would be cool if it shows up, but if it doesn't there's always another possibility..." With dreams there is no 'how'. Dreams have an energy all of their own and when you follow the flow of that energy, your dreams come true, as if by magic. Dreams usually don't include winning lotto... that's mostly a fantasy!

What's interesting is when we look at creating our own reality, we create a fantasy reality because we don't believe we can have what we truly desire. If you want to create a dream rather than a fantasy, look at what you desire and ask: "What would it take to have this?" Then stop and be quiet! Let the universe provide the awareness of what is next. You will know when you know! Forcing it will not create knowing (but it will create anxiety, stress and a sense of missing out!) Using your knowing is the principle of "BE first, DO second" in action. It is a simple way to allow harmony between your inner world and the possibilities in your outer world.

Knowing is instantaneous and feels like space. You can have that feeling walking down the street — you don't need to hide in a cave meditating for 30 years to have inner knowing! Knowing is intuitive awareness for busy people... Would you be willing to use your knowing to take the shortcut to flow? Remember, if it feels light it is true for you... if it is heavy you may want to make a different choice! Would that create way more fun and ease for you?

A great question to play with when you think you don't know is "What do I know here that I don't know I know?"

And then allow your knowing to show up, no force, just flow!

With every choice we are inviting the future into form. What we choose in this moment creates new possibilities. Does what you are being or doing in this moment have the potential to create your dreams? If not, you may want to make a different choice.

The care and nurturing we create this moment with impacts the future too. We think of being powerful as making something happen. But what if it is really about being aware of where we can put our energy so that our reality can be changed? Everything has energy. What happens when we ask that energy to support our dreams and visions? What happens when we are willing to ask for everything and not have a point of view about what shows up? The universe can always deliver more than we imagine possible.

BURNOUT
BREAKTHROUGH ACTION

The biggest changes are often created from the smallest of questions. Doubt is not a question. It is the answer we use to stop ourselves from having full awareness of what is possible! Judgment is not a question. It is the tool we use to eliminate possibilities and keep ourselves the same as everyone else.

Here are some of my favourite questions:

What creative energies can inspire me today?

What can I create that no-one else can?

What creative possibilities are available to me right now?

What creative edge can I bring to this project?

What creative capacities do I have that I haven't been using?

INSPIRATION
& INSIGHTS

Do you have a fantasy that you could create awesomeness in the world without being different, without standing out, without stepping into the possibilities that come your way? I know you're trying not to be 'too different', but this unwillingness to acknowledge your true magic keeps your burnout in place. When you have all your focus on what's wrong with you, you have to keep trying to fix you, rather than being the creative adventurer you truly are (even if that seems like an idea from another planet right now.)

By the way, if you're going to dream big, sitting in front of a computer can limit your awareness. I do a lot of my big thinking and exploring of energetic possibilities at the beach and on mountaintops because I love the sense of spaciousness and peace. If that's not possible then a nice comfortable chair and some tactile creative notebooks are great for capturing the essence of what's next.

DEVELOPING CREATIVE ROUTINES

Your creative self is buried deep under a lifetime of habits and beliefs. When you gently peel them off, you discover this raw, real you that is curious about the world and intrigued by the creative energies you have access to. So, how do you develop creative routines that keep you alive and thriving, rather than just going through the motions of living?

Routines sound boring, and yet they are the building blocks of creating ease. Being a naturally creative person (even when it was well hidden under a pile of burnout), I had strong resistance to any sort of routine — it just didn't sit well with me and so I was always lurching from one forgotten mess or half-finished project to another — until a very insightful friend said "be creative in your routines and routinely creative".

These few words have changed my life — I no longer resist routines that I can make creative. For example, for me, grocery shopping is much more joyful at farmers markets than in a supermarket. Paying my bills is totally blissful when I playfully ask the money to return to me a thousand fold!! Cleaning the house is easy when I use it as a purposeful time of moving meditation — being in the moment and enjoying the results of my creative inspiration as I rearrange and make beautiful as I clean.

PAUSE. BREATHE.

SAY YES.

Here are a few areas where it is beneficial to have a creative routine in place.

- Food shopping … eg food markets, cooking new recipes, making healthy treats!

- Cleaning the house… sexy it up with funky music or make it a meditative experience.

- Set a place for 'dumping' stuff when you walk in the door… and a place for leaving stuff you need to take with you! (You'll never spend 10 minutes looking for your keys again — I promise!!)

- Movement… do what makes your body feel amazing, not what everyone says you should do. If you don't like moving, get a dog and make your movement playful!

- Starting and ending your day… when you have creative clarity, your day will run more smoothly! (Check out the free Morning Magic e-class at www.LivingBeyondBurnout.com/morning)

Neuroscience is now proving what creative geniuses through the ages have always known. Routine can unlock the door to creative inspiration, IF it is a creative routine!

- Boring routines produce uninspiring work; creative rituals allow for the spontaneity that produces awesome work.

- Boring routines ensure life is predictable and safely dull, creative rituals allow for the richness and diversity of life to emerge gracefully.

- Boring routines feel like an imposition or habit that is unchangeable; creative rituals bubble up from inside you in surprising ways, making each time a fresh experience!

- Boring routines create busyness; creative rituals allow you to ask questions that enhance productivity.

- Boring routines distract you from what's truly important; creative rituals allow you to discover the magic inherent in purposeful great work.

- Boring routines help you cope with chaos; creative rituals allow you to flow with life's challenges in unexpected ways.

- Boring routines take you out of the present moment and out of your body; creative rituals allow you to be intensely present and fully aware of your intuitive knowing!

As you can see, it is not just any old routine that needs to become a habit... creative routines create the space and connections which allow magic to unfold in all sorts of unexpected ways.

Creative routines are the catalyst, the trigger and the signal to your BEing that you are now freeing yourself of your duties, your challenges and your distractions... because nothing is more important in this moment than allowing yourself the freedom to be who you truly are and create something of value for yourself and others.

No genius ever delivered great work from a space of stress, stagnation or the status quo!!

Creative self-expression is important to sensitive people. Whether it be in creating a calm, nurturing environment or one that draws you out, a physical expression of who you are is a great reminder when your mojo is missing in action. You know how it works, those gorgeous heels create a confident persona you can slip into... that jacket takes you into the corporate war zone, allowing you to escape unscathed... those funky jewels give other people like you a visible point of connection and conversation.

PLAYFUL IS THE NEW MINDFUL

Imagine there are only two ways to live. You can put all of your attention and creative energy OUT into the world, being led by the people, ideas, projects that take your fancy. Or you can intensify your internal creative energy so much that it overflows into the world and everyone *including you* receives more.

In the first one, you become distracted, depleted and it destroys your future as your creative energy is constantly dissipated in trying to connect with the world.

In the other, you become potent, playful, pleasure-filled… and it creates your future, as your creative energy feeds you so much creative inspiration that you change the world by who you be.

I contend that playful is the new mindful. Have you tried being mindful? Have you tried being playful? Which one works best for you?

If your work isn't working, you can change yourself or change the spaces you are playing in. You can change the physical space, the energetic space or the emotional/mindset space you operate in. Creating change in any of these spaces will create the possibility of new choices and new perspectives.

When we are in an authentic space that feels right to us, nothing can stop our light from shining on the world. When we are out of play (literally!) that feeling of flow can be more flighty and indefinable than a butterfly on a warm summers day.

BURNOUT
BREAKTHROUGH ACTION

There are moments in each day (that can turn into hours) when you unexpectedly find yourself with 'free' time. Maybe a meeting is cancelled. Maybe you find yourself suddenly home alone. Maybe you are waiting for someone. Maybe you are too tired to do anything that requires a brain.

Instead of pushing ever forward on a treadmill filled with the next 'to-do' or 'to-create', invite yourself into the space of a nurturing creative retreat. Receive the gift being offered to you and stop running so fast. Breathe. Give yourself a moment to wonder. Allow your being to become present with your body. And then ask... what kind of creative retreat could I gift myself right now?

You could colour-in, doodle, knit, decorate a corner of a room, write a story, paint glorious watercolour sketches, explore which of your ideas may like to have idea babies... there are a thousand possibilities! (If you need more inspiration, check out my 'Stop Waiting, Start Creating' book at www.StopWaitingStartCreating. com) I like to carry a tiny creative kit with me - what's in it varies, but it means I always have a means of creative expression.

Enjoy the moment, allow your spirit to be replenished and allow your life to flow.

INSPIRATION
& INSIGHTS

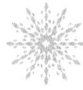

HUSTLE LESS,
FLOW MORE

There's one story that too many of us have bought as real, that is responsible for a lot of unnecessary burnout. It's this: "Hustle is good. Hustle is essential. You can fix everything by adding hustle." No, you can't... and it's not. It's an energy born in the ghettos of struggle and stress, and we don't need more of that in the world.

Hustle is force, aggression, push and moving fast. It implies scarcity. It invites a continual hunger for more that cannot be satiated, or if it is, you're judged as being complacent or lacking ambition. It's competitive and actively turns up the 'fight or flight' energies in your body which lead to adrenal exhaustion. It is the opposite of flow. It's held up as the solution for getting everything, and yet, it shows up in our lives as an insidious and particularly nasty form of grinding misery that saps the life out of you. Hustle is a resistance to timing, a resistance to being and a resistance to collaborative, co-creative contribution. If you want to mess up your life and intensify your burnout, just add hustle.

When you are in flow with your life, hustle isn't necessary. When you are rested and relaxed, you are in a space of receiving. Living joyfully brings ease to you! Now, I know this sounds like a fairytale when you're in deep do-do and you think the only way out or forward is to go harder, be more productive or perform better. If that was going to work, you wouldn't still be in the do-do. It would have changed your situation by now. So, this is where your unwinding begins.

Before burnout your body gives you a whole lot of more subtle hints about what is not working. It might be tired, or resisting a particular project, or getting you to meet people who have different ways of creating. Your body is phenomenally smart - whether or not you listen to it! Burnout comes from forcing yourself to keep going in the face of those sweet little whispers and inklings, rather than going "Hang on a minute, something's not right here, what needs to change?"

Working 24 hours a day on something you couldn't solve working 12 hours a day won't change it any faster. Working 12 hours a day when you function a thousand times better working only six hours a day is crazy. And we've all done it! Why? Because it's easier to fit in than to say no, or to take a mental health day off, or to look underneath the surface at what is really going on. It's easier to fill your life with work than fill it with pleasure when you are making the struggle real.

PAUSE. BREATHE.

CHOOSE.

DO SOMETHING DIFFERENT

If you want to create a different way forward, you have to do something different. What got you here, won't get you there. Today, it starts with giving up the hustle. "Hurry up and get what you want," is an exhausting way to live. When you ease up on the constant doing, you'll have enough space to perceive with clarity the exact choices that allow everything to move forward with greater ease. This doesn't mean you have to function like a tortoise, just that you have to allow enough space to be aware of everything that IS available, before you act. It's elegance in motion!

Whenever I'm in 'do-do' land and I have a big list of stuff to get through, I often start by going to the beach for a few hours. Why? Because those few hours create the clarity that makes that list easy to move through. If you don't have a beach handy, there's plenty of other choices - play with your pets, go for a walk or run in nature, lie in a park and watch the birds, do some painting or art... anything that is playful, gives you space and engages your body so that your mind can stop thinking will work! One thing — when you're in the play-zone, don't actively think about your list... clearing your mind is the start of having ease instead of hustle.

When you stop making hustle greater than you, your body can show you another way forward. Trauma and stress dissipate with nurturing, calming responses, not intensification of the strain. How can you bring the energy of flow into your world? It might be as simple as watching a surfing video, knitting or scribbling big wavy lines. The process is more important than the result. I painted walls (very slowly) for the first few weeks after I left my job because that rhythmic movement was allowing my mind to unwind. It needed that space to let go of the stress and trauma so that I could put together a coherent sentence once again.

Flow is interrupted when we make time relevant, when our environment is not supportive, when we spend our energy on trauma and drama rather than self-care, when we don't have the support we need to live with ease, and when we are disorganised and lacking systems. These elements are the foundations of flow. Do you allow the space for building your foundations or do you resist it and skip straight into putting the roof on, even though there's nothing available to hold it up?

Since leaving the corporate world I've not worn a watch. If I need to know the time, I have my phone. I prefer to live and create outside of time. Time is a construct and it's only relevant because we make it so. I tried so many time-management systems, none of which made any difference to my life. When I began seeking an unconventional solution to the non-stop hustle, it came in the form of energy management. When I am acutely aware of how I'm using my energy, there is space for everything to come to fruition, often in unexpected ways. One way out of the hustle is to manage your energy. Do what makes you feel good, as often as you can. Follow your intuitive knowing and it will show you non-linear shortcuts. You'll have more energy and the clarity will come!

MANAGE YOUR ENVIRONMENT

Your environment needs to support your wellbeing. Declutter. Make it beautiful. Make it functional and comfortable. This may include removing some people from your world. Who is a contribution? Who is a hindrance? What conversations need to be had to create more ease and flow in your daily life? Who can you add to your life that will support you and contribute to greater possibilities? You don't have to know right now, but start asking for new people to play with. One thing I always ask for is people who love ease and flow and who are willing to have it. So much trauma and drama leaves your world when you invite playmates and workmates who value ease! And then your energy is used for fun, rather than fixing everything and everyone.

What systems do you need for your life to run smoothly? What are the 'problems' or challenges that you repeatedly deal with? Start with those, they need a system in place so that there is ease going forward. Design the system to create a greater possibility where flow and ease are paramount, rather than just fix the surface level issue that keeps presenting itself. This applies to your body, your life and your work!

Having your foundations in place provides a magical platform for flow to be available on demand. I love writing, but I noticed my writing was intermittent at best. So I created a regular writing hangout where a group of us get together online and write. Oddly enough, these three hours of sustained writing have paved the way for me to make writing a daily priority. One choice can be the catalyst for new ways forward. Even if I only write for twenty minutes, I value making space for writing each day. Making that small commitment means I wake up most days with awareness of a topic ready to be explored - I've asked for this ease and the universe delivers the flow.

One last thing... have you noticed it's so much harder to be in your brilliance when your focus is hustle? When you invite flow, your brilliance is naturally and intensely present. You don't have to try. You don't have to prove. You just have to be (you!). Say goodbye to hustle... listening to your awareness is the antidote.

BURNOUT
BREAKTHROUGH ACTIONS

1. Ask a question - "Universe, can you show me how to have ease and flow with this please?" and then be responsive when new possibilities show up in your world.

2. Leave space for doing 'nothing'. That space creates the magic you think hustle will give you. I promise!

3. Follow the energy when you are inspired.

(Check out www.LivingBeyondBurnout.com/inspire for my interview on how following the energy works in daily life.)

INSPIRATION
& INSIGHTS

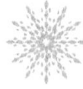

4. TURNING UP YOUR BRILLIANCE

BRILLIANCE IS YOUR SECRET SAUCE!

"There is nothing in a caterpillar that tells you it is going to be a butterfly." ~ Buckminster Fuller

Allowing your brilliance to shine seems like an incredibly odd way to transform burnout. If you had asked me to do that when I had burnout, I would have imagined you were a little unhinged. All I really wanted was to feel better. Don't talk to me about brilliance! In hindsight, I wish someone had had the conversation with me that I'm about to have with you. But first, a little of the backstory on 'why brilliance?'.

The last time I had burnout, it started during a relationship with a narcissist. Realising that burnout could come from other places besides my work, I started searching for bigger patterns. I discovered that every time I had burnout, I was not being everything I am. I was not being true to myself. I was not allowing my brilliance to shine, or I was allowing it to be bullied out of me. So not pretty!

In contrast, when I looked at the times in my life when I've had the most energy, when I've been happiest, it has always been when my brilliance was in full flow. In these situations, I was not obsessively proving myself, not being a stitched-up perfectionist, not preoccupied with responding to other people's expectations and projections. Instead, I was joyfully, wildly in my creative flow. I was using my talents and still discovering more. I was at ease in the world as I was trusting my awareness and allowing my brilliance to shine, without doubting it.

Here's the moment where you may be wondering... "Well, why wouldn't you just be like that all the time?" I wondered that too! I realised that as a highly sensitive (aware) person, I am always acutely aware of my environment. Acutely aware of all of the people, how they are functioning, what they need, what they desire from me. What was missing in the burnout situations was a sense of myself. I had become lost in other people's worlds, without the boundaries that would allow me to function at my best.

If you're in the midst of burnout and the physical symptoms are stopping you in your tracks, you're probably wishing that your body would have the energy to deal with even 10% of your brilliance. You are probably more than slightly frustrated or depressed that your body is failing you in your quest to do everything.

SHUT UP. I'M NOT BRILLIANT.

If you're thinking "Shut up about the brilliance! I'm way too exhausted to even consider the possibility. And if I really am as brilliant as you're saying, how did I get stupid enough to get burnout?" I hear you. I was stunned to realise I could be that smart and that dumb all at once!

In order to defend your burnout and defend against your brilliance, you first have to judge it as right (or wrong). What if you could open your awareness to the possibility that burnout and brilliance are far more closely intertwined than you desire to know... what contribution could that be to the creation of a very different future? One where YOU are more valuable than anything you deliver or create or do. Creating a fun, adventurous life and a nurturing business or career need not be filed under 'impossible unless I'm perfect first'.

ACKNOWLEDGE THE BRILLIANCE YOU'RE PRETENDING NOT TO HAVE

So where do you start? You stop being the moth to the flame. You stop singeing your wings in attempting to prove you're brilliant and you allow your brilliance to be there, whether anyone sees it or not. The only opinion that matters right now is yours. Do you truly acknowledge your own brilliance, or are there always a few sneaky doubts heckling you from the back row of your stadium, undermining everything you seek to create? When you acknowledge your brilliance, it allows your full presence to shine. You don't make anyone greater than or less than you, and yet, you are totally clear that you are what you are. It is not other people's acknowledgement and approval you seek, it is your own.

We have a night sky full of reminders of our brilliance. We are made of stardust. Shooting stars are the sparks of brilliance that explode into being when you stop controlling them. When you fully embrace your brilliance, you will shine non-stop, effortlessly. Until then you live in the darkness of your unspoken dreams, illuminated only by the random bursts of genius you can no longer contain.

Imagine your world if you stopped burning out your light... if you stopped containing yourself by exhausting your body... if you stopped being less than what you truly are. Is it a different world? For me, burnout has always been about change. It is my very clever body's way of saying 'Hey you, I know you think you're in charge, but you're not listening to me, and you can't go far without me! I know stuff too!'

ACKNOWLEDGEMENT ISN'T BOASTING

What does it take to turn up your brilliance; to fully embody the presence that allows the world to know your brilliance exists, so that others may also be inspired to choose more? The willingness to be superior with no apology or hiding. Being superior is different to doing superiority.

'Being superior' is acknowledging your brilliance and contribution in its entirety, without turning into a gloating smart-ass who has to prove and prove and prove their superiority. When you are superior, you quietly know that your contribution makes a greater difference in the world than most people are willing to consider, let alone make. This unspoken awareness offers an undefinable and irresistible invitation to everyone in your sphere of influence to discover and embrace their greatness too.

When you acknowledge your brilliance it allows you to receive the contribution of others - without having to have everything be perfect, or for you to be the only one who can create and do things. You get to give up being an overwhelmed over-achiever, in favour of being the brilliance that will magnetise other brilliant people towards your flame, so that you can all shine brighter together. You can stop doing everything alone and stop exhausting yourself by proving that you can do everything. There is no proving involved in being superior; you just get to BE the magic and brilliance of you!

PAUSE. BREATHE.

ACKNOWLEDGE.

'Doing superiority' is a judgement. It's where you are pretending to be brilliant and you are constantly deciding who is in/out and what is 'the best' for everyone and everything. It is not an invitation to create more; it creates the possibility for people to feel 'less than' rather than embracing their brilliance in its entirety. It invites competition, confusion and the kind of disconnection that shows up as bullying, abuse and being an asshat. I sense this is not exactly what you were aiming for when you started being an over-achiever.

When you have an acute sense of awareness, it is confronting to choose to be superior. You don't want to stand out in case it brings you more of the same misery that you've spent your life trying to avoid. And yet, it is this same awareness that can open the doors to truly living. Being an aware, potent presence that can change the world by your unconventional, unpredictable choices.

Here's an example of how this plays out in real life.

I have a verdant capacity for talking about the elephant in the room. To me the energy of the unspoken is stronger than an elephant's memory and just as vivid. When I talk about what I sense, it freaks people out because they thought those things were hidden. If I am being superior, I'll be aware of the effect of what I'm about to say before I say it — and I'll choose whether or not to say it based on the future it will create. If I am doing superiority, I'll put the cat amongst the pigeons (or the elephant among the chickens) without a second thought as to the impact on other people and the future. The first comes from being aware, the second comes from proving. When you give up proving your worth, your brilliance becomes a trillion times more valuable.

To acknowledge how brilliant you are, you have to be generous with you. When you are generous with you, you put you first. This doesn't mean you're selfish. It means you stop doing everything for everyone else, at the expense of you, so that they are all comfortable and happy, even if you aren't. Has it occurred to you that if they aren't choosing joy and ease, they may not want to have that as their life? Who gave you your superhero's cape? Or did you pick it up at 7–11 on your last 'save the world' mission? Maybe the world isn't asking to be saved. Maybe it's asking for a totally different possibility. You can't lead it there if you're suffering from the need to fix everything and everyone without being asked. Besides which, fixing things is a slow train to oblivion.

Right now you may be squirming a little. It's uncomfortable to see the dark side of your brilliance and it's even more uncomfortable to own your brilliance. Amongst all of this, you definitely won't allow yourself to settle for being mediocre. It is this conflictual paradigm that has you shuffling around the dark, draughty halls of burnout — unfulfilled, unengaged, unhappy. How much longer are you going to choose to avoid the brilliance that is the doorway to all possibilities?

WHAT IS BRILLIANCE?

Your brilliance is everything you are aware of that others don't even notice. It's everything you sense that others do not perceive. It's the difference you are, and the weirdness you're trying not to be. Brilliance is everything you are when you're not trying to fit in with other people… or 'get it right', or prove yourself. Brilliance is being fully present in your aliveness, your awareness, your vulnerability and openness, your potency and power.

- It is intuitive intelligence — tapping into your awareness rather than working everything out with your mind.

- It is being open — receiving from others, being you and being vulnerable, rather than being a 'power over' kind of leader.

- It is being creative — rather than being bound by habits and routines

- It is presence with what is — rather than wishing for what is not currently available.

- It is being curious and allowing possibilities to expand — rather than limiting yourself to the known.

You were not born stupid or slow. Your superpowers are hidden under layers and layers of lies. Otherwise identified as dusty old points of view projected at you by people who were terrified of your brilliance. Seek the people who build you up, who acknowledge your contribution, who see your true capacities. Let go of the people who are always showing you how to be less, or who keep putting you in situations that stifle your innate creative potency. And most of all, make a promise to yourself that you'll never dim your light for anyone.

Your brilliance is luminous. You are a luminary, albeit a tired, joyless one right now. What would it be like to embrace this brilliance, welcome it and allow it to show you the contribution it can be to enlivening your life.

BURNOUT
BREAKTHROUGH ACTION

Find a beautiful notebook or journal. Before you go to sleep each night, write a love-note to yourself. Include in it five ways you were brilliant today. You are brilliant at least 900 times a day and 1001 of those times you do not acknowledge your genius, instead you negate it and you in the cruellest of ways. If you'll start to acknowledge your authentic contribution, it can expand. As it expands, you'll have more energy. (Yes, it is this simple!!)

Oh... and one more thing. Start with a fairly loose interpretation of brilliance. Don't set the bar so high that you've got nothing to admire about you. I promise, you'll thank me for this for the rest of your life.

If you never stopped your brilliance again who would you be? What would you be? Where would you be? Take a moment to explore this... and make a promise to yourself to turn yourself up, not off, as you face the world.

INSPIRATION
& INSIGHTS

HOW DO YOU STOP YOUR BRILLIANCE?

It's useful to know the ways you stop yourself. I didn't see many of these until they were pointed out to me. This is not an exhaustive list… it's an invitation to discover exactly what it is that you allow to hold you in the throes of burnout.

How much energy does it take to dumb yourself down to match the energy and awareness of the stupidest people around you? When you make stupidity real it uses a lot of energy. How much of your exhaustion is due to choosing to be less than who you truly are? Ever found yourself making any of these choices? They may be the exact things that are making you ridiculously tired!

1. *Buying other people's points of view about you as real and true.* Seriously? You value those people's opinions above your awareness? All judgement is designed to stop you. What if none of those perspectives are anything to do with your reality? No-one knows you like you do! Trust you.

This one is tricky. We're trained from school-age to believe other's judgements of us. The thing is, they see you from the outside only. They cannot know what is inside you. But you do. Value that. Grow that. Love that until it shines so bright and so clearly that the dirty smudges of judgement become irrelevant.

2. *Cutting off your awareness of what you know, because it doesn't fit the dominant perspectives.* When did you stop being the leader you truly are?

Did you ever have a brilliant idea, look around, see that no-one else is doing anything like it, and then decide your idea must be useless? What if it's not? If Einstein, Edison, Marie Curie, Elon Musk and Richard Branson had done that, the world would be a very different place. It's exhausting to only create basic ideas when you have genius ideas coming to you. Playing small looks bad on you. Stop it!

3. *Making yourself as slow and stupid as the people you care most about, or spend the most time with.* They may be loveable, but you don't have to make yourself less to love them or have them love you.

At school, I was the slowest runner imaginable. And brilliant in almost every other way. It took me years to discover that I'd (unconsciously) made myself slow physically so that I wouldn't be too much for the people around me. By being not so athletic, I found a way to sort of fit in, even though I was a misfit in almost every other way. As I got older, I realised that I couldn't talk about how fast I was, that I didn't really need to study, that so many things came easily to me, because people didn't like it. And then I realised that never acknowledging this was stopping me from creating even greater. Is there somewhere in your life you have a similar story? Is it time to upgrade your choices?

4. *Sharing your brilliance with those who can't receive it limits the impact of your brilliance, especially if you are not willing to be as totally weird and different as you are.* Sometimes brilliance is 'just for me, just for fun… never tell anyone'. How weird are you that you've never admitted to anyone, including you?

When you celebrate how weird you are, people's opinions have no power. Charles Dickens. Johnny Depp. Russell Brand. Madonna. Lady Gaga. YOU! They don't let small-minded people stop their creative genius and so they don't get worn out by the stupidity of people who think small and normal. When you let people make your weirdness wrong, you become less. It's hard to be small when you're born to be big. I know showing up feels like the last thing you want to do right now. So start by showing up for you. It's a muscle. Build it.

5. *Not being creative or showing your brilliance in the world because you don't want people to steal your ideas.* Is it worth stopping you to stop them? Or can you just keep out-creating them and keeping them guessing as to what you'll do next?

Charles Dickens' biography described the many times he lost control of his publishing rights and watched other people make a lot more money than he was for his creations. He never gave up, he kept negotiating new ways forward and he never made his competitors significant. His target was to be the greatest writer of his time and he always had something new up his sleeve, both creatively and legally. Is it possible you have some kind of brilliant, creative capacity too?

6. *Pretending that you only have the choices that other people have.* What if your particular brilliances offer you far more choice than other people are aware of? Are you only going to make the choices that they can see? Or will you start using your gifts for you?

If you desire to disrupt an industry, you have to know you have different choices. Look at JK Rowling - she has totally disrupted what it is to be an author by making choices that other people don't have available. You have choices just as brilliant as hers, but you don't make them because you're too busy being less than what you are. I know it sounds harsh, but it's part of what creates burnout. You need to see where you're fucking yourself over. This is the tough love section. Funnily enough, if you find the courage to choose different, you'll thrive gloriously in every moment instead of dying a thousand small, painful deaths every day.

7. *Trying to be brilliant in the ways other people are.* They must be right... right? Rather than being brilliant in the ways YOU are!

We all know this one a little too well. It looks like comparing your inner world with everyone else's outer world. It looks like wanting to be what someone else is, while constantly ignoring the brilliance of you. It looks like being less magic than you are so that you can fit into a linear, logical paradigm that has nothing to do with how you actually create.

PAUSE. BREATHE.

BE AWESOME.

OWNING YOUR BRILLIANCE

In case no-one has told you this today, you are awesome, just the way you are. Your crown has been ready for you since birth. It is your choice to wear it or leave it gathering dust in a corner. You can polish each jewel or let your brilliance be dulled by your disinterest. You can nurture your brilliance gently, or let it get bent out of shape by allowing everyone who comes along to prod and poke at it. Your crown is not a crown of thorns. Your crown does not exist to tell others who you are. It is a reminder to you that you are a powerful, glorious, sovereign leader with many brilliances that can be played out in the world. Will you adore and explore your brilliances as joyfully as you would the gold and precious jewels found in your crown? Or will you continue to hide them, as if being brilliant is something to be ashamed of?

If you were one of the smarter kids in your class at school, did you ever feel like you should hide it in some way? That your brilliance was intimidating for the people around you? If you weren't academically smart, you may have been brilliant in other ways… ever been in trouble for being funny and making everyone laugh? Or have you always been aware that what people were saying and what they really thought were two different things?

I have a dear friend who has been convinced that she is stupid. No matter how many times I told her that I wouldn't be able to hang out with her if she was, she would not believe me. She was taught she was stupid at school, because she didn't fit the so-called 'normal' learning patterns that schools offer. Her brilliances are in non-traditional areas and so, for most of her life, have been unacknowledged, even though she has been hugely successful both financially and in raising her family.

It is a wondrous thing to watch someone emerge from their cocoon. Will you look in the mirror and allow yourself this gift? No-one except you can unhook you from the judgement that you are stupid. You have to stop believing what other people say.

You cannot let anyone else judge you or define your

brilliance. Your brilliance goes far beyond intelligence. How many people do you know who are hiding their brilliance and doing everything in their power to get you to hide yours too, so that none of you have to come out of the darkness and be who you truly are? This is how we've created the dumbing down of our society. What would it be like to be so generous of spirit that you celebrate brilliance in all its forms?

What if you were so phenomenal and so potent that you could be a million times more effective than anyone around you? What if you were willing to be the gift of sensitivity (awareness) to everyone around you? What could you add to their lives and businesses? What could you add to your own life and work?

Most sensitive people beat themselves up for everything that is 'wrong' with them, rather than recognising what is right about them that they aren't getting! So, what is right about you that you aren't receiving?

Too often we are taught that we have to suffer first before we can have the rewards that will transform us... The caterpillar endures extreme struggle to morph into the beautiful butterfly. Without the struggle, the butterfly's wings do not unfold with strength and purpose. You can choose the caterpillar route if you want to... personally I'd rather be a dolphin! Somehow using your strengths with ease and joy sounds like a lot more fun! If you've accidentally turned on caterpillar mode, explore the Burnout Breakthrough below. Your ocean of possibilities is calling!

BURNOUT
BREAKTHROUGH ACTION

Make a list of all the ways you imagine you are 'wrong' or 'less than' others. Ask yourself where the brilliance is in each of these spaces. And then ask "What talent do I have that would allow me to be this brilliant?" It's time to stop working so hard at life and business! Instead of watching Wonder Woman and wishing for superpowers, start acknowledging the ones you have that you aren't yet using.

As Access Consciousness® founder Gary Douglas asks 'What if your wrongness is your strongness?' As you discover the brilliance in each of your 'faults' or 'weaknesses', you set yourself free to be everything you are – at full capacity, not as the smallest, most shrivelled-up, most exhausted version of you!

INSPIRATION
& INSIGHTS

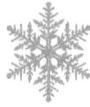

LOVING YOUR WORK

"We are all here for some special reason. Stop being a prisoner of your past. Become the architect of your future." — Robin Sharma

Your work can energise you and expand your creative capacity in the world, or it can diminish your energy, leading you towards burnout. You don't have to quit your job like I did. There are gentler transitions available. I hope this book has found you a little earlier in the process and you are stopping the downhill slide so that you don't land at rock bottom.

This chapter invites you to look at your work with fresh eyes. Take an hour or two in a quiet space to begin exploring your work. Especially if you aren't enjoying it.

What is working? What is not working? Is the situation changeable or do you need to choose a new situation? If you move into a new role, identify the underlying changes that are will make the greatest difference so that you aren't faced with the same situation again, just in a different environment. Our personal habits and choices have much more of an influence on what's possible than we acknowledge.

The saddest conversations I have are with people who think they must put up with a less than optimal situation. There is always choice, even if it doesn't appear that way on the surface. Dig deeper. Get extremely clear on what you desire to have as your work-life, and start taking steps toward it. Find ways to add joy and play to your daily work.

If you have duties you detest, ask if there is another way for those things to be done. In many of my jobs I negotiated to have someone else do the things that were not in my zone of brilliance. Often that work would end up being done by someone who loved it — the change made both of us happier! We are all different for good reason. Make the most of your differences and you'll contribute to other people having new choices and adventures too.

PAUSE. BREATHE.

REFRESH.

LOVING YOUR WORK STARTS HERE...

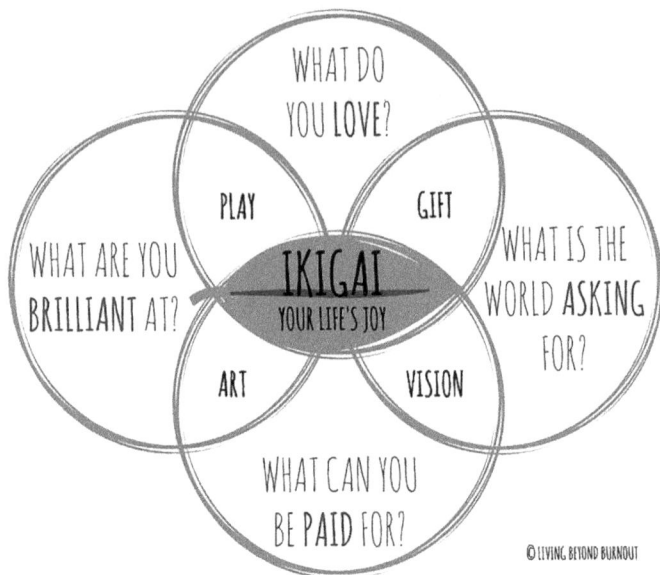

WHAT DO YOU LOVE?

PLAY

GIFT

WHAT ARE YOU BRILLIANT AT?

IKIGAI
YOUR LIFE'S JOY

WHAT IS THE WORLD ASKING FOR?

ART

VISION

WHAT CAN YOU BE PAID FOR?

© LIVING BEYOND BURNOUT

The Japanese word 'ikigai' is loosely translated as the 'the fruits of living'. It includes all that makes your life worth living, and it invites your true possibilities to blossom. When your work delivers ikigai, it offers you a joyful, blissful adventure, rather than being a drudgerous energy-zapping theft of your time.

Loving your work starts with play. Play is found at the intersection of doing what you love and what you are brilliant at. When you are focused on your brilliance, you can let go of being perfect. You are enjoying the journey in every moment, rather than being obsessed with the destination. Brilliance opens the doors to work being play. How can you bring play into your work today? If you aren't sure, re-read the Creative Energies section.

When you intensify your brilliance and allow yourself to be paid generously for it, your unique magic turns into art. You bring who you truly are into the world at the highest levels. This doesn't mean you need three post-graduate degrees and a host of industry awards. It means you show up every day as the brilliance you are. And you offer that brilliance with so much love and generosity that people know they can count on you for the most intriguing perspectives, the most interesting ideas, the most creative ways forward. When you make what you do into art, you become a leader worth following. Being in demand brings financial rewards. Be open to receiving money — whether it is for a side-gig or it is your main source of income. Money expands the choices you have available.

In the space where what you love and what the world is asking for collide, you get to be the gift you came here to be. You get to contribute your energy to the world in useful ways. You get to receive feedback from the world that your gift is valuable and makes a difference. This is the area where deep personal satisfaction emerges. When both you and others receive bliss from what you love, it is energising.

The bountiful mix of what the world is asking for and what you can be paid for is where your vision begins to strengthen. What is the change you are inviting others to choose? What are the possibilities that only you are aware of? What choices do you have? Your vision embodies the creation of future possibilities in profitable ways. Your vision determines your priorities. When you stop saying yes to everything, you'll be able to say yes to the choices that will be the greatest contribution to you and the world.

Now… if you are in the midst of burnout, you may be too exhausted to even think about changing the world. But, as we discussed right back at the start of Section Two, change and choice are a fast-track for making your symptoms disappear. Not as a way of adding 'more to do', as a way of changing the way you live and work, so that it is more aligned with who you truly are. Starting where you are allows what is 'not you' to dissipate and disappear… and that frees up a whole lot of energy!

BURNOUT
BREAKTHROUGH ACTION

Right now you may not even be clear where you are. Using the descriptions and an outline of the model above, draw your personal treasure map of what you are aware of right now in relation to the play, art, gift and vision that is relevant to you. Use dot points, add stories, aha moments, ideas you are curious to explore... start to see the patterns that already exist. There is no right answer here, it's an exploration of possibilities.

It is going to be tempting to write down a heap of not so happy things — do yourself a favour... don't write them down unless you can turn them into a strength. For example, back in the burnout days, if you'd asked me what I was brilliant at, I would have sarcastically responded 'exhaustion'. The upside of exhaustion is being able to choose change... I am great at change; I'd just missed the memo that said 'change now'. Where is the strength in your wrongness? If you seek strength, you may be surprised at how it shows up!

INSPIRATION & INSIGHTS

FOUR ELEMENTS FOR CREATING IKIGAI

1. WHAT DO YOU LOVE?

To love your work you may need to make changes. Your choices include negotiating a different way of working in your organisation, changing jobs internally or externally, starting a side-gig or starting a new business. The following questions are a way of exploring what works for you. This is where a lot of career direction books start and stop. It's also where the lie 'do what you love and the money will come' tends to originate. Joseph Campbell said 'follow your bliss', he didn't add 'and the money will come'. He knew that when you choose this, magic shows up. It is not a linear or logical process.

For example, I love painting. I once painted for ten days straight even though I was supposed to be working on a thousand deadlines. At the end of that time, I realised that those paintings were the basis of my new brand imagery, which I hadn't been able to envision with ease. It never shows up how you imagine it should. So… do what you love, and allow it to show you the way forward.

Loving your work is one of the best antidotes to burnout available. I don't mean that obsessive kind of love where you won't let go of your babies (that's not actually love!), I mean the pure, innocent kind of love where each choice you make enhances the pleasure and experience of living. Where your heart is so fully engaged that you have a sense of joy and bliss in each action you take.

What you love comes from sources far beyond work. It includes people, pets, leisure activities, adventures, sport, travel, playing games, energies, nature… and so much more. What did you used to love that you've forgotten about? What did you always want to love, but haven't yet explored? What makes you happy? What makes you relaxed? How can you bring these energies into your work?

- What kinds of jobs or environments have allowed me to be my best self?

- What kinds of bosses or workplace culture allow me to show up greater than I imagine I am?

- Where is joy most present in my work? Where can I be more present with the joy?

- Where is creative play most available in my work? If it doesn't exist yet, how can I add it?

The biggest question for me in loving your work is 'how do you prefer to work'? When you know that you work best early morning, or in twenty minute bursts, or in complete silence (or with heaps of white noise) you can start to set up your environment to make your work pleasurable.

The how is just as important as the what... and right now, you may have more control over the how than the what. Seek to change what can change with ease. Each choice opens up new doors for future choices. If you can't immediately make the quantum leap to how you best work, say yes to every tiny choice that moves you forward.

2. WHAT ARE YOU BRILLIANT AT?

Before you say 'nothing' remember that every single one of us shows up on this planet with the gifts and talents that we need to live a full and joyous life.

- What do I naturally know that other people don't?

- What comes so easily to me that I find it crazy that other people don't get it?

- What energises me effortlessly?

- What do other people praise me for (when I'm feeling well)?

Getting clear on your brilliance is not about comparing yourself to others, or lying to yourself so you can feel better. It's about deeply acknowledging the essence of you that you came here to enjoy, indulge in and offer to the world as your gift.

Brilliance often shows up in our darkest moments or through our greatest challenges. I had no idea I could write with more ease than 99.99% of the earth's population. Being able to write was what got me through my MBA. Without that gift, I would not have been able to complete it whilst in the midst of burnout. Even under the greatest physical duress, words still came. Maybe not as fluently as before, but they didn't desert me. Speaking was another matter entirely - the circuits between my brain and my mouth took a much bigger hit than the circuits between my awareness and my hands. Weird!

Right now, what is it you can still do, even though you feel like death warmed up? What is the challenge or theme that repeats itself in your life? How do these elements connect with your brilliance? Whilst the answers may not be obvious just yet, if you keep asking for the connections to be visible, you will discover the brilliance that has been hidden until now.

One last comment... your brilliance resides in your heart, rather than your mind. Don't seek it through thinking; allow it to emerge from your being.

3. WHAT IS THE WORLD ASKING FOR?

Your particular mix of brilliance offers something the world is asking for. Whether you deliver it through a job or by starting a business doesn't matter. What matters is identifying what it is that you can gift to the world.

For me, this special gift is 'choice'... having people know that they don't have to live in limited ways. Offering playful ways for people to discover that there are many ways forward, and none of them involve the energy of 'should'. Inviting people to create new possibilities, rather than living in the 'must dos' that society dictates. How did I come to it?

When I first quit my job, I had become so insular that I had no idea what the world was asking for. Hell, I didn't even know what I was asking for, besides a new body! (Which is not a great ask by the way... sometimes the Universe gets literal!)

For about two months, every time I went out, I made it a game to explore what the world was asking for. I'd eavesdrop in cafes; I stalked advertising signs; I listened for what people were complaining about; I explored what I desired but could not find in readily available forms. I looked for gaps where I could make a difference. Through this process I made a list of 300+ ideas. Not because I thought I'd create them all. I just wanted to have choice!

- What is missing in the world?
- What is asking to be changed?
- What would make the world a more fun / happier place?

As I explored different ideas, I made notes on what was available at what price. I also talked to people who were selling things I found interesting. How did they get into that type of work? Was it working for them? What were the downsides? What did they most love about it?

All of this research gave me a sense of possibilities. From the bones of the research, I started a couple of businesses which I quickly discovered weren't right for me. It didn't matter; they were experiments that took me closer to what I was seeking... which was far better than staying in a job where I was suffering.

What most clearly defined my path forward was looking closely at the patterns of when I most loved my work, and when I most hated it. What were the defining characteristics of each?

- What was I contributing when I was happiest?
- What was I not able to contribute in the situations where I had burnout?

- What contribution could I see was needed in the world, but completely lacking? What skills did I have that could create this?

Exploring these questions gave me a clear sense of what was important in how I would interact with the world going forward. Then it was time to look at how I could be paid for what was fun for me!

4. WHAT CAN YOU BE PAID FOR?

This is the question that you may be freaking out about, especially if you've had a regular paycheck for a very long time. Relax. You don't have to give up your job, but you may want to start a side gig that gives you more satisfaction. Or find a way to bring your brilliance into your main job. Is there anything your employer needs that you would LOVE to offer them? Maybe part of your recovery from burnout is swapping some of your normal duties for a special project?

If you have your own business, you either know what you can be paid for, or not knowing is part of what is creating your burnout. I discovered what people would pay for with a whole lot of experiments (that I continue to create because they are fun for me!)

There are many ways to find out if people will pay for your expertise and magic. The first is to ask them — "If I offer xyz, would it be useful to you? If so, how much would you be willing to pay to solve or change this situation?" is a simple way to start the conversation.

Another way to find out if you can get paid for what you love is to research how other people are getting paid for similar ideas. You may be surprised at what is possible. One word of warning — just because someone has a flash website, doesn't mean they are making money from their idea. Your research may need to go a little deeper.

- What can I get paid for that is so outrageous I've never considered it until now?

- What do people try to pay me for that I refuse?

- What did I used to get paid for that I loved?

- What are other people getting paid for that makes me slightly envious?

The other element you need to consider here is what are you willing to be paid for? For many of us, when people offer us money for things that are incredibly easy, we almost feel like a fraud for taking the money (so much so that some people refuse to take the money at all). This is the insanity of the world we live in. If our work is too easy, there is so much judgement for making money from it, when the reality is that a happy world would be one where everyone makes money with this much ease. You don't get paid for the struggle or challenge. You get paid for your energy and insight. Receive the money graciously, and don't hide what is easy for you, as if it has no value.

PAUSE. BREATHE.

LOVE.

MY VISION

This chapter started as a separate book that may one day also be published — I'm not sure yet! It evolved through a strong desire for every person in the world to be able to do work they love and be paid well for it. Can you imagine the level of happiness that would be created if every person on the planet had this choice? There would be no more burnout!

In this moment, my dream may seem far off, but every person who chooses this possibility shows others how to access the choices that lead to loving your work. Every leader who ensures their teams are doing the work they are most brilliant at enables more joy at work. When we play with this together, a new reality becomes possible.

BURNOUT
BREAKTHROUGH ACTION

Explore the questions in this chapter (listed here for your convenience)... just one or two at a time. Go deep. Be honest with yourself. What do you know that you don't admit to yourself or the world? Is it time for a new future?

1. What do you LOVE?

What kinds of jobs or environments have allowed me to be my best self?

What kinds of bosses or workplace culture allow me to show up greater than I imagine I am?

Where is joy most present in my work? Where can I be more present with the joy?

Where is creative play most available in my work? If it doesn't exist yet, how can I add it?

2. What are you BRILLIANT at?

What do I naturally know that other people don't?

What comes so easily to me that I find it crazy that other people don't get it?

What energises me effortlessly?

What do other people praise me for (when I'm feeling well)?

3. What is the WORLD asking for?

What is missing in the world?

What is asking to be changed?

What would make the world a more fun / happier place?

4. What can you be PAID for?

What can I get paid for that is so outrageous I've never considered it until now?

What do people try to pay me for that I refuse?

What did I used to get paid for that I loved?

What are other people getting paid for that makes me slightly envious?

INSPIRATION
& INSIGHTS

SECTION

III

CREATING YOUR
GREATER FUTURE

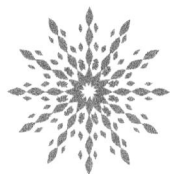

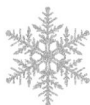

CREATING YOUR
GREATER FUTURE

By now you've realised there are a few unconscious choices going on in your life that no longer work for you. Soldiering on. Trying harder. Creating through force. Fixing everyone else's problems. Resisting change. If what you've been doing isn't working, it's time to change the channel! You wouldn't keep listening to a radio station full of shitty songs… so don't keep living a life full of shitty choices.

The predictable choices that everyone expects you to make take you away from the present, away from what IS possible right now. You are in a transition time. It may mean taking some space for you. Slowing down rather than running faster and harder on the treadmill that never stops.

You only have one limitation.
Not choosing the change that is possible.

The journey of transition from exhaustion to energised creates a much deeper transformation than you may expect. It can be instant or take you lifetimes. It depends how much resistance you have to starting and changing.

Did you ever drive somewhere? Did you wait for all the lights to turn green before you left the house? Or did you leave, knowing that you're fully equipped to respond to whatever situations you discover along the route?

When you choose change, the tiniest choices can shift your energy in an instant. Right now, you can start by choosing one of the four themes we've covered in this book. Commit to making a difference in the easiest ways available and allowing everything to shift as you keep choosing what lights you up. Here they are again…

Change… creates a difference in the space and nature of daily living.
Creativity… creates bliss for the spirit.
Nurture… creates ease for the body.
Brilliance… creates adventures and achievement for the mind.

I know you'd love to logically choose where to start. What if that's not the easiest way forward? Nature rarely moves in straight lines. By making logic king, human nature attempts to stop the chaos which creates true greatness. Chaos is not havoc. Chaos is the energy nature uses to create new realities.

Instead of choosing logically, write those four themes on separate pieces of paper, screw them up, mix them around and ask your body to choose which one will be of greatest benefit to you today. Then play with the Burnout Breakthrough Actions from those chapters.

You can also discover additional ideas at www. LivingBeyondBurnout.com/insight.

There's also a fun quiz at www.LivingBeyondBurnout.com/ quiz that will give you simple ways to get started, based on where you are at right now.

When you bring the energies of change, creativity, nurture and brilliance together, you create harmony and ease in your living. You may also have other ways of expressing your mind, body, spirit and life… don't limit your choices to these themes, use them as a springboard for discovering the future that is seeking you.

When your energy comes back and you feel great again, it's tempting to go back to your old habits. Please don't!

These four elements from the Burnout Breakthrough Model

are now a daily part of my life. While I keep them in harmony, the burnout beastie is kept at bay. If I accidentally move into workaholic mode, or highly sensitive and not coping mode, the burnout symptoms can make themselves known quite quickly. I've discovered those old ways of living are better kept in the past where they belong.

The future we are creating now is about being alive and thriving. Living in harmony with our body. Enjoying our creative energies and allowing our full brilliance to shine.

Anyone can be a workaholic. Not everyone can be brilliant, successful, playful and relaxed. You make yourself mediocre by making the choices that everyone else can make. When you make the choices that only you can make, you create the change you are seeking beyond your wildest dreams.

DON'T DO THIS ALONE!

I have a gorgeous friend who was Buddhist and burned-out. When she went to the bank to get a housing loan they refused it because, according to her beliefs, she told them the truth - that she'd had a nervous breakdown and her income had decreased as a result.

No-one wants to admit to burnout or a breakdown because of archaic responses like this. It's time for all of us to create a different future.

What kind of world have we created where you are shamed and disadvantaged for being truthful? Ultimately, when you tell it like it is, it sets you and the world free, and it's clear the path to that possibility is still being formed.

In speaking up, you invite new ways forward. You discover it's not you that should be ashamed. The society we have created is fast to judge and slow in its generosity. Whichever part you play, would you be willing to work together to create different ways forward?

PAUSE. BREATHE.

LEAD.

I highly recommend keeping a journal of the change and choices you create. Share the aha moments, the breakthroughs, the choices that work for you. Allow others to know there is a way forward, and that having burnout doesn't have to be a shameful secret.

As you start recovering, encourage open discussions in your workplace. Bring the experience of the themes we've talked about into your daily work with your team and colleagues. Open the doors to burnout being preventable, rather than an expensive and extreme recovery mission.

When we create this possibility together, the world will change. Imagine a world without burnout. A world full of people who love and adore their work and their life in true harmony. A world without hustle. A world where creative flow is recognised as the most productive possibility. This is what we are creating.

If you'd like to be part of this awakening, join the Amplify Your Energy Lounge at www.AmplifyYourEnergy.com

BURNOUT
BREAKTHROUGH ACTION

CREATING YOUR FUTURE WITH EASE
AN ENERGY IMMERSION

You can create a totally different future if you choose.

Listen to this energy immersion via audio here:
www.LivingBeyondBurnout.com/inspire

You are looking across a river and on the other side is all the energy you desire. Up until now, you've spent your entire life trying to solve the problem of how to get to the other side - and being angry and frustrated that no matter what you do, you can't seem to find the way.

You try lots of things, but none of them seem to work and you get more and more angry. Other people feed your anger by being angry with you and for you. You start thinking you are doomed to always fail, and, instead of building a bridge, you build an anger mountain. Whenever you seek an answer, the anger mountain responds, clouding your awareness and stopping you from knowing what would work for you.

One day, you decide to give up being angry and frustrated and you throw yourself in the river, allowing your body to float effortlessly downstream.

On the way to the ocean, your awareness shows you how to move towards the river bank you have been so longingly seeking for such a long time. Instead of being angry that you don't know the way, you embrace the flow and you start to trust that you will have everything you require to get there.

As you enjoy the flow, you get closer to the opposite shore, sometimes it reaches out and touches you! And then one day, you find your feet standing firmly on the shore of being fully energised.

How did you get here? In removing your anger goggles and refusing to be frustrated by your situation, you made the space to begin receiving the thousands of tiny and not so tiny hints the universe had been trying to send you. As you responded to the flow of those hints with curiosity and a willingness to create something totally different, the river moved you to all of the places where energy and thrival are available to YOU.

Maybe yours isn't an anger mountain - it might be a resistance mountain, or a struggle mountain, or a fear mountain, or a doubt mountain, or a depression mountain... whatever it is for you, know that you can change it by making just one choice. That you won't allow your life to be ruled by that energy mountain any more.

And then throw yourself into the stream of living and begin to receive everything that is available to you through your awareness...

It's not about deserving, or being a good person, or doing things perfectly or any of the thousands of excuses and judgements we put between us and having an ease-filled life.

When you welcome your intuitive awareness with not a single barrier, the river is always flowing. Wildly throw yourself into the current, let go of control and receive the whispers.

There. Is. No. How.

Awareness. Is. The. Real. Magic.

*** You can use this energy immersion in many ways. Swap out what YOU desire for *energy* and insert your specific obstacle as the mountain and you have the way forward for creating pretty much anything you desire. Have you had enough of pretending to be a muggle? ***

INSPIRATION
& INSIGHTS

BEEN THERE, DONE THAT, READ THE BOOK… NOW, WHERE DO YOU START?

That's a great question! Let's ensure overwhelm does not become your best friend again. Start by being present with what is right in front of you. I found I was only miserable or unable to cope if I was in the past, or worrying about the future. In the present moment, you have everything you need. Start where you are.

Download a summary of the Burnout Breakthrough Actions for easy reference at www.LivingBeyondBurnout.com/insight

Thank you for joining me on this adventure in Living Beyond Burnout. There is much to discover about living your best life. Thank your burnout for setting you clearly on the path!

My life now is a trillion times greater than I ever imagined possible. And there is still so much more magic to come. I'm beyond grateful to the burnout for opening my eyes to the limited life I was living. For showing me that hard work is not the way to living brilliantly. For ensuring that I would seek new ways of creating success in business and life.

What can you be grateful to your burnout for? What futures can you create that you've never even considered? Gather your courage, your life is beginning anew.

Trust your brilliance. Trust your magic. Trust your creative essence. These energies are the start of your phenomenal new life.

ARE YOU SEEKING MORE?

Throughout my burnout adventures, I received contribution from many people. Please know you don't have to do this alone. There are many ways to be supported. These are the things I offer, and there are many other people that can also contribute to your wellness.

If you would like to take this journey with other people in similar situations, I offer live support in the *Amplify Your Energy Lounge*. Find out more at www.AmplifyYourEnergy.com Together, we rise.

If you would like me to do a media interview, speak at your conference or for your organisation, please contact me via my main website: www.CreativeAlchemi.com

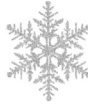

REFERENCES

INTRODUCTION

Aron, Dr Elaine.The Highly Sensitive Person. Available at http://hsperson.com/https:/www.amazon.com/Highly-Sensitive-Person-Thrive-Overwhelms/dp/0553062182. Last Accessed on November 13, 2017.

SECTION 1

ARE YOU LIVING WITH BURNOUT?

Stillman, Jessica. 2017. "The 12 Stages of Burnout, According to Psychologists" in Inc.com August 02. [Originally published: Kraft, Ulrich. 'Burned Out', *Scientific American MIND*. June 2006.] Available at: https://www.inc.com/jessica-stillman/the-12-stages-of-burnout-according-to-psychologist.html. Last Accessed on November 10, 2017.

Parker, Madalyn. 2017. Twitter Status Update. June 30. Available at: https://twitter.com/madalynrose/status/880886024725024769. Last Accessed on November 10, 2017.

LIBERATING THE REAL YOU

Csikszentmihalyi, Mihaly (1992) '*Flow: The Psychology of Happiness*'. Available at: https://www.amazon.com.au/Flow-Psychology-Happiness-Mihaly-Csikszentmihalyi-ebook/dp/B00GO8HZIW. Kindle New Ed Edition 2013. Ebury Digital.

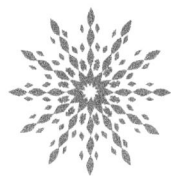